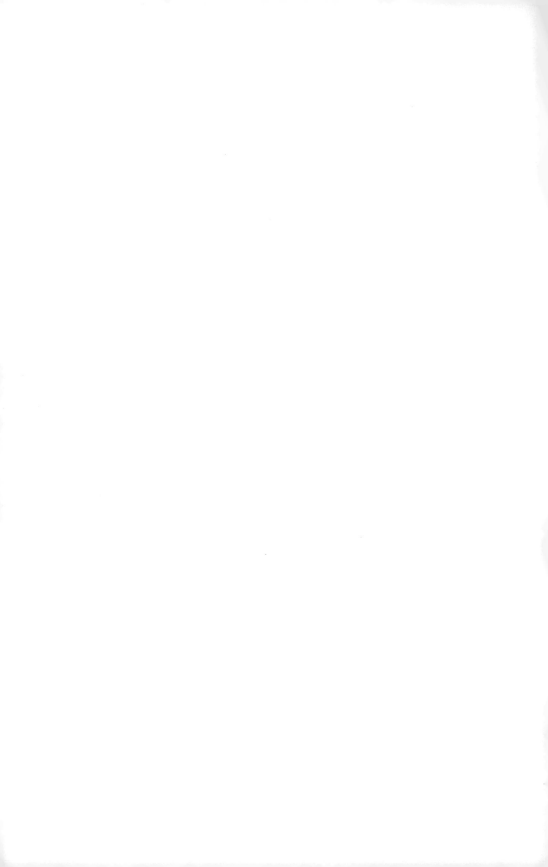

Encyclopedia of Autism Spectrum Disorders

Volume II

Encyclopedia of Autism Spectrum Disorders Volume II

Edited by **Paul Spencer**

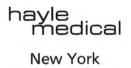

New York

Published by Hayle Medical,
30 West, 37th Street, Suite 612,
New York, NY 10018, USA
www.haylemedical.com

Encyclopedia of Autism Spectrum Disorders
Volume II
Edited by Paul Spencer

International Standard Book Number: 978-1-63241-123-5 (Hardback)

Contents

Preface

This book extensively discusses Autism Spectrum Disorders (ASD) and its related aspects. Many researches are being conducted in the field of ASD and substantial efforts are being made to study it. It is usually difficult for any professional to keep pace with the current developments in this field. This book includes contributions of expert clinicians and renowned researchers from all over the world. It aims towards providing latest information and advances in the area of ASD. It gives broad overview of the topics which may be unfamiliar to researchers and clinicians. The topics have been organized under three sections: etiological factors – co-morbidity; sensory issues, alcohol syndrome & relationships and etiological factors - parents & family.

This book is the end result of constructive efforts and intensive research done by experts in this field. The aim of this book is to enlighten the readers with recent information in this area of research. The information provided in this profound book would serve as a valuable reference to students and researchers in this field.

At the end, I would like to thank all the authors for devoting their precious time and providing their valuable contribution to this book. I would also like to express my gratitude to my fellow colleagues who encouraged me throughout the process.

Editor

Aetiological Factors - Co-Morbidity

Pre-Existing Differences in Mothers of Children with Autism Spectrum Disorder and/or Intellectual Disability: A Review

Jenny Fairthorne, Amanda Langridge, Jenny Bourke and Helen Leonard

Additional information is available at the end of the chapter

1. Introduction

The autism spectrum disorders (ASD) represent a group of severe and chronic neuro-developmental disorders often simply referred to as autism. [1] Using the criteria provided by the *Diagnostic and Statistical Manual of Mental Disorders, Fourth Edition*, ASD are diagnosed by impairments within the three strands of DSM-4: *social interaction, communication* and *repetitive behaviours or interests*. [2] The aetiology of autism is complex. [3] Research has implicated a strong genetic basis [4-7] involving multiple genes [5, 7, 8] and possible gene-environment interactions. [9-13] Advances in chromosomal microarray analysis and gene sequencing technologies have improved diagnoses and suggest that aetiologies of ASD will continue to be uncovered. [9] In addition, a child presenting with autistic symptoms may be found to have a certain genetic mutation which accounts for their true underlying biological diagnosis. For example, a diagnosis of Rett syndrome would be confirmed when a girl with ASD and intellectual disability was found to have a mutation of the *MECP2* gene on the X-chromosome. [14] Children with ASD and intellectual disability have been found to have an expansion of the *FMR1* gene confirming a diagnosis of Fragile X syndrome. [15]

Autism and intellectual disability commonly coexist with 30-80% of persons with ASD reported as also having ID. [16, 17] Currently, the relationship between ASD and comorbid ID is poorly understood. [18] However, it is known that phenotypically, persons with these disorders can be grouped into the three categories of ASD without ID, ASD with ID and ID only. [18] Intellectual disability (ID) is characterized by an intelligence quotient (IQ) of less than 70 which is associated with limitations in at least two areas of adaptive skill and which is manifest before 18 years. [19] The level of ID is generally grouped into the five levels of mild, moderate, severe, profound and unspecified by IQ score. In research it is common to stratify ID to the following three levels defined by the American Psychiatric Association [2] (Table 1).

Descriptor/level of ID	IQ score
Mild or moderate ID	35-40 up to 69 points
Severe or profound ID	< 35-40 points
Unspecified ID	< 70*

*Here the person has been assessed as having ID but has not been assessed adequately to determine the level.

Table 1. Levels of intellectual disability

In terms of aetiology, ID can be broadly divided into cases of known biomedical cause and those of unknown cause. The biomedical causes may be divided into genetic and non-genetic causes. Further subdivisions are given in Figure 1.

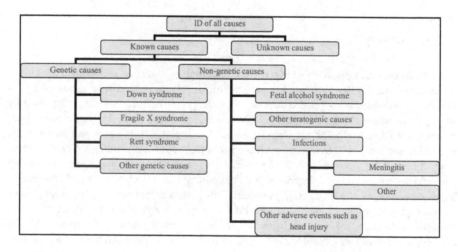

Figure 1. Commonly known aetiologies of intellectual disability

In addition to genetic and non-genetic causes of ASD and ID, relationships with socio-demographic factors such as a mother's education, [20, 21] immigration, [17, 22] and ethnicity, [23] have also been identified. Other reported associations involve aspects of a mother's health including physical characteristics [24] physical [25, 26] and mental health [27, 28] and health behaviours. [29, 30]

It has also been reported that milder autistic traits are present in other family members of individuals diagnosed with ASD. This phenomenon has been coined the Broad Autism

Phenotype [31] and includes qualitatively similar, but milder traits in areas such as language, personality and social behaviour. Some researchers believe that identification of the Broad Autism Phenotype in family members might provide a complementary strategy for detecting genes which contribute to the likelihood of ASD. [32, 33] When comparing family members of a child with ASD to persons from the general population, subtle differences within the Broad Autism Phenotype could be associated with specific brain regions, particular neural pathways, and ultimately with particular genes. [33]

The above factors have been used as guides in choosing terms for our literature search to examine pre-existing characteristics of mothers of children with autism and mothers of children with intellectual disability of unknown cause. Inherent characteristics of mothers of children with a specific disability could be associated with the genetic, environmental or genetic-environmental aetiology of their child's condition. It is therefore important to separate pre-existing factors, particularly in relation to mental health, from morbidities such as depression [34] which might develop due to the more intense demands of caring for a child with ASD and/or ID.

The aim of this study is to review research on the pre-existing characteristics which differentiate mothers of children with ASD and/or ID of unknown cause from each other and from mothers of children without these disabilities. Such an investigation may help to further clarify the determinants of ASD and/or ID including the role of genetic and modifiable risk factors. Improving our understanding of the genetic and environmental causes of ASD and ID may reduce the future burden of these disabilities [35] by hastening the development of effective prevention and treatment strategies.

2. Literature search and selection

The papers considered for this review resulted from a search of the Medline, Web of Knowledge, Scopus and Google scholar databases. Combinations of the search terms below were chosen.

- Terms associated with ASD and/or ID: autis*, pervasive development disorder*, intellectual disability, mental retardation, disab*;

- Terms associated with ASD and/or ID aetiology: immigra*, migra*, ethnic*, age, socio-demographic, prenatal, perinatal, auto*, immun*, anti*, psych* and phenotype*; and

- Terms associated with mothers of children with ASD and/or ID: traits, characteristics, parents, mothers, children, persons.

A paper was included in the review if:

- It was accepted for publication between 1st January 1990 and 31st October, 2012 inclusive;

- It was a full text article in English;

- It described new research and was published in a peer-reviewed journal;

- It described the results of a cohort, case-control, correlation or cross-sectional study of at least 15 subjects;

- It compared a characteristic of parents or mothers of children with ASD and/or ID with parents or mothers of children without disability or with a population norm;

- It assessed characteristics that were pre-existing and not likely to be a result of caring for a child with ASD and/or ID; and

- It used methods of ascertainment and measurement of the characteristic(s) of interest that were assessed as unlikely to lead to bias.

Eighty papers were retained for the review. We stress that these papers do not represent the entire literature pool in the area. Had we chosen different search terms or used different combinations of terms in our searches, the basis for our review would possibly have been different. The three categories for our analyses were; *socio-demographic factors, immigrant status and ethnicity* and *health and physical characteristics* and we sorted papers by these categories. An additional 61 articles were used to provide background information and possible explanations of some of the reported associations.

3. Socio-demographic factors

There are a number of considerations which impinge on the effect of socio-demographic factors on the prevalence of ASD and/or ID. Firstly, in persons with ASD with ID and those with just ID, the features overlap to some degree. A child with ASD with ID, particularly in the past, may often have been diagnosed with only ID as there have been secular changes in the identification of children with ASD. Secondly, persons who could be diagnosed with ASD without ID are most often able to function independently and may remain undiagnosed in a range of scenarios. Thirdly, the process through which children are assigned a diagnosis of ASD is much more complex than for ID. Whilst elsewhere, the gold standard might be the considered judgement of an expert clinician who had seen many patients with autism [36], in Western Australia, a diagnosis of ASD in a child requires an assessment by a team comprising a paediatrician, psychologist, and speech pathologist. Waiting times for this assessment can be prolonged in the Western Australian public system [37] and even longer in the US. [38] One effect of these considerations is that in some countries a child whose parents are socioeconomically disadvantaged may oft times be diagnosed with ID when a diagnosis of ASD could be more appropriate.

3.1. Socio-economic status

Thirteen articles researched the parental socio-economic status (SES) of children with ASD and/or ID [17, 20, 21, 39-48] and all but two [42, 43] supported a different association of SES with ASD than ID. Children with ASD were more likely to be from higher SES families but children with ID were more likely to be from lower SES families.

A range of measures of high SES were consistently associated with ASD. In a large telephone interview study in the US, family wealth was used as a measure of SES. [40] The researchers found that children from higher income families were more likely to have a diagnosis of ASD. Similarly, others using family income as a marker for SES, found a significant association between high family SES and ASD in the offspring. [47] Further analyses, using the dual markers of high family income and high maternal education, found a particular association between high SES and ASD without ID. [47] Using population data and deriving SES from mother's place of residence at time of the child's birth, Australian researchers also found that ASD, ASD with ID and particularly ASD without ID were associated with higher SES. [17]

The overall association between high SES and ASD without ID could result from the increased empowerment of parents of high SES to pursue a diagnosis where their children have a milder variant of ASD. [49] In families of low SES, higher functioning children with autistic traits might be informally labelled by family and contemporaries as unusual, difficult or emotionally damaged. In a comparable way, lower functioning children with autistic traits might be formally or informally given a diagnosis of ID. Others have suggested that children of lower SES parents might be more likely to be diagnosed at a later age than those of higher SES and hence not be included in studies of ASD and SES with lower ages of cut-off. [49]

Further evidence of the possible social contributions to the likelihood of an ASD diagnosis was found in a large multi-based national study in the US. [39] Undiagnosed children who met the criteria for ASD had a lower SES than children who had been previously diagnosed. [39] Area-level SES indicators derived from census data were used in another study where the researchers elucidated that increasing SES and the increasing prevalence of ASD were associated in a dose-response fashion. [39]

King et al. [41] provided evidence that an interaction of social factors was affecting the likelihood of an ASD diagnosis. They examined factors influencing the likelihood of an ASD diagnosis using data on around five million births in Californian cohorts from 1992 to 2000. They found that an interaction between high and low level SES measures influenced the likelihood of an ASD diagnosis. Medi-Cal is a program providing medical assistance to the needy in California and these researchers used family use of Medi-Cal as a binary measure of SES. Property values in the area of a mother's residence were also used as a measure of SES. These researchers reported that children whose families were enrolled with Medi-Cal births and living in wealthier neighbourhoods were two and a half times more likely to receive a diagnosis of ASD than their counterparts living in poorer areas. [41] This could indicate that for parents of limited resources, living in a higher SES neighbourhood had benefits in terms of the likelihood of their child being diagnosed with ASD. Possibly, this results from the parents' increased access to support persons such as paediatricians and child health nurses and to educational programs such as parent classes and interventions for children, compared to that of similar parents in less affluent areas.

In contrast, a Danish study accessing linked population data, used maternal education and parental wealth as a measure of SES and found no association between SES and ASD diagnosis. [42] In neighbouring Sweden, a population-based study published in 2012, used low income, manual occupation and less education as measures of low SES. The researchers concluded that low, not high SES, was a risk factor for ASD. [43] There may be a number of reasons for the differing findings of these studies. The universal health-care and routine screenings offered in

Denmark and Sweden may eliminate the ascertainment bias associated with high SES which may exist in other Western countries. [43]

By comparison with ASD, low SES was often identified as a risk factor for ID [21, 44-46, 48] and especially mild or moderate ID. [17, 20, 48] One of these studies was a cross-sectional study of over five million children. [48] It concluded that children with mild or moderate ID had an increased risk of exposure to social conditions which were detrimental to their development. [48] Another study examined SES and ID prevalence in the 1966 and 1985-6 Finnish birth cohorts. [46] The researchers concluded that the association of low SES with ID was present in both cohorts. Plausible hypotheses for this persisting association are that there had been no improvements in antenatal and obstetric care in those of lower SES over the twenty years in question or, alternatively, there is a prominent genetic involvement in the aetiology of ID. Another, is that the higher risk of exposure to a developmentally unfavourable environment has persisted over the 20 year interval in the children of mothers of lower SES. [48]

In total, ten studies [20, 21, 23, 41, 45, 47, 50-53] used education alone as a measure of SES. All four of the studies investigating ASD reported positive associations between high maternal education and the risk of ASD in the offspring. Three of these studies were from California and each reported that parents of children with ASD were more educated than the general population. [21, 41, 50] The fourth reported that mothers with more than 16 years education were more than twice as likely to have a child with ASD without ID than mothers of a child with only 12 years education. [47] The relationship was reversed with maternal education and ID where all research ascertained a negative association between high maternal education and the risk of ID in the offspring. For instance, with children with unspecified ID [20, 21, 23, 45, 51, 53] and developmental delay without ASD [24](which may include those with known genetic syndromes), seven studies concluded that their mothers were of a lower educational status. One of these, a population study, established that mothers of children with ID were less likely to have more than 13 years of education. [23]

The association of maternal education with varying levels of ID has been investigated including for severe ID and on the basis that risk factors for Down syndrome differed from those of other forms of ID, children with Down syndrome were excluded. Mothers of children with severe ID were found to be more likely to have a lower educational status than mothers in the general population. [52] Comparable results were found for mothers of children with mild or moderate ID [20, 21] of unknown cause. These mothers had increased odds of a lower educational status than mothers in the general population. One of these studies used Californian service agency records and a sample of more than 27 000 mothers of children with mild or moderate ID or severe or profound ID. [21] Less maternal education was also associated with an increased risk of severe or profound ID in the offspring.

3.2. Marital status

Four papers, describing five studies, examined marital status in relation to the odds of ASD and/or ID. [17, 20, 46, 54] At the time of their child's birth, it is uncertain whether a woman's marital status is associated with her odds of a child with ASD. However, mothers of children with ID were more likely to be without partners.

In Australia, a retrospective cohort study, using linked health registries assessed marital status in terms of living with a partner. They reported that at their child's birth, women living with a partner were 35% more likely to have a child with ASD and particularly ASD with ID. [17] On the other hand, a similar Canadian study found that mothers not living with a partner at the time of their child's birth were 19% more likely to have a child with ASD than those mothers who were living with a partner. [54]

With ID, women without a partner had increased odds of having a child with ID [17] and particularly mild or moderate ID. [20] Similarly, a cohort study using UK data, concluded that compared to typically developing children, those with early cognitive delay were less likely to have their biological parents living together during the first five years of their lives compared to families with a typically developing child. [55] However, in Finland, the negative association between living with a partner and the odds of ID in the offspring, present in a 1966 birth cohort, was absent in the 1985-6 cohort. [46] The reduction of the association in the second cohort may have been a reflection of the improved SES of single mothers over the 20 year period.

3.3. Parental age

In most studies, increasing maternal age, sometimes along with increasing paternal age, was associated with ASD. A minority of studies found relationships only with paternal age or found no association with either maternal or paternal age. Contrasting results were reported with ID where teenage mothers were more likely to have children with mild or moderate ID were older mothers and particularly likely to have children with severe or profound ID. Socio-demographic and biological explanations are offered.

All ten studies investigating the association of maternal age with the prevalence of ASD found that advanced maternal age was associated with an increasing prevalence of ASD [17, 29, 47, 56-61] and sometimes ASD without ID. [17, 47] Four of these studies, reported an additional association with paternal age. [17, 56, 58, 61] For instance, a population-based study using data from multiple sites throughout the US, found associations with both maternal and paternal age after adjustment for the other parent's age, birth order and maternal education. [58]

Five of the cited studies specifically reported an association between paternal but not maternal age and ASD in the offspring. [58, 62-65] One of these studies was a small Japanese case-control study of 84 father-child dyads. The researchers reported that advanced parental age was associated with nearly twice the risk of ASD without ID. [65] Another was a population-based Israeli cohort study which used data from a medical registry. [63] The remaining studies used population data from Sweden and another, population data from Denmark. [62, 64] After an adjustment for maternal age, the Swedish researchers identified a linear association of increasing paternal age and the risk of ASD. These researchers commented that if no adjustment was made for paternal age it would appear as though maternal age, rather than paternal was the risk factor for ASD. They added that paternal age could be a risk factor as generally the male was considered to be the origin of new mutations in the gene pool and their production increased with age. [62]

By comparison, three studies from Northern Europe, and UK identified that neither of advancing maternal nor advancing paternal age was a risk factor for ASD. [42, 43, 66] One of the studies from Denmark and another from Sweden used linked data from national registries. [42, 43] The third was a much smaller UK study of around 5 000 participants and parents provided data by completing self-reports. As with broader measures of SES, the results from Denmark and Sweden might reflect the model of health service provision in Scandinavia. Moreover, there is evidence that children with ASD are diagnosed later in younger mothers. [67] Thus there may be a bias of ascertainment in some studies where younger children are included. In the UK study, [66] younger mothers may been included more often since they were recruited when pregnant. Further, a diagnosis of ASD was not required for their child but instead, a parent completed the *Social and Communication Disorders Checklist*. In other studies from the US, [41, 47, 58, 59] Canada [29] and Australia, [17, 57] ASD may be under-ascertained in the children of younger parents, possibly as a result of their lesser confidence to be pro-active in the diagnostic process.

Maternal age had a dual association with ID of unknown cause. Firstly, teenage mothers were more likely to have children with mild or moderate ID. [17, 20, 21] Secondly, older women were more likely to have children with severe or profound ID. [21, 68] The results of a Finnish cohort study which investigated ID of both known and unknown cause [46] was discounted because of the inclusion of ID of known cause. With Down syndrome, the most common cause of ID, it is known that the risk increases very abruptly with advancing maternal age. [69] This might explain the researchers' finding of an association between increased maternal age and ID in the offspring seen in the 1966 birth cohort. [46] The finding that the association no longer existed in 1985-6 cohort may have been because of the introduction or increased uptake of prenatal screening for Down syndrome.

The association of parental and particularly maternal age with ASD and/or ID suggests that both social and biological forces are operating. Younger parents may find a diagnosis of ASD more difficult to obtain for their children because of inexperience and navigational require-ments of local systems. Thus, some of the ID diagnoses of their children may be undiagnosed cases of ASD. Further, the excess of older mothers of children with ASD and to a lesser extent ID may result from increased de novo mutations in older women and their partners [70] or the increase of epigenetic mechanisms which are associated with ageing. [71]

3.4. Parity

Parity describes the number of live-born children and stillbirths at more than 20 weeks gestation of a woman. [72] Two strong relationships of low parity with ASD and high parity with ID have been demonstrated in the majority of studies.

In women of lower parity, the risks of ASD, [29, 41, 73] ASD with ID [17] and ASD without ID [17, 74] were found to be increased in a number of studies. One of these was a Canadian cohort study using linked data-bases and with nearly 1 000 case mothers. [29] The authors identified that nulliparous women (that is women having their first child) were at the greatest risk of having a child with ASD. Moreover, a national, population-based study in the US reported that older nulliparous women with older partners were around three times more likely to have a child with ASD. [58]

However, two studies found other associations between parity and the risk of ASD. The first, a Danish case-control study nested in population data, found no association. [42] The second, a prospective cohort study using linked health data of more than 110 000 mothers in the US, asserted that mothers of parity greater than two were more likely to have a child with ASD than other mothers. [25] Possibly, socio-demographic factors were also operating in this circumstance. In relation to SES and the odds of ASD, it is possible once again that the disparate findings of this same Danish study may have been due to less ascertainment bias which set them apart from other studies in the area. [42] The second study involved nearly 120 000 nurses who were followed via their completion of mailed questionnaires over sixteen years. [25] Hence, all mothers were educated and due to their involvement with nursing, could be expected, on average, to have more knowledge of ASD than other mothers. Further, parity was assessed as a binary variable with the two values of greater than two and less than or equal to two. Commonly, other studies have defined parity as either a continuous variable or one with more than two possible values and this difference might account for variations in study findings.

Mothers of higher parity had increased odds of having a child with mild or moderate ID. [17, 20, 21] One of the research groups concluded that fourth or subsequent children had an increased risk of mild-moderate ID. [20] A Finnish study of two birth cohorts, twenty years apart, found that high parity persisted as a risk factor for ID over time. [46] A large cohort study compared the parity of the mothers of Californian children with ID to the parity of mothers of typically developing children born between 1987 and 1994. [21] These researchers reported that mothers of parity of three or more were 30-50% more likely to have a child with mild or moderate ID or unspecified ID. [21] Both this study and another Californian study reported that mothers of children with severe or profound ID had an elevated but not significantly increased parity compared to mothers of typically developing children. [21, 52]

3.5. Summary

Socio-demographic factors often operate quite differently for ASD and ID. For example, high parental SES was positively associated with the risk of ASD and negatively associated with the risk of ID in the offspring. Marital status, as defined by living with a partner, has different associations. At the time of their child's birth, there was no consistent association of marital status with mothers of a child with ASD compared to the mothers of typically developing children. On the other hand, mothers of a child with ID were less likely to be living with a partner than mothers of typically developing children. Parity appeared to have reverse associations for ASD and ID. Compared to mothers of typically developing children, mothers of low parity were more likely to have a child with ASD and mothers of high parity were more likely to have a child with ID. Similar patterns exist for maternal age. Mothers of an advanced age were more likely to have a child with ASD than mothers of typically developing children. In contrast, mothers of a younger age were more likely to have a child with ID than mothers of typically developing children. However, an additional association exists with older mothers being also more likely to have a child with severe ID.

An under-ascertainment of ASD due to social factors and, to a lesser extent an over-ascertainment of ID could be contributing to the socioeconomic effects seen with ASD and ID. For instance, in terms of the severity of ASD, researchers in California, with birth cohorts from 1992 to 2000, divided the children with ASD into two groups of equal size where the less severe group comprised children in the top 50% of cases according to level of functioning and the most severe group was the lower 50%. [41] They found that the children from the less severe group were more often found in neighbourhoods which housed wealthier and more educated individuals. Conversely, the same researchers reported that where low SES was measured by a Medi-Cal payment for the birth, the ratio of more severe to less severe cases was always greater than one. The researchers' interpretation was that the most difficult to diagnose cases of ASD, that is the less severely affected, were under-ascertained in lower SES populations. [41]

The association of high SES with ASD also might be compounded by some of the characteristics known to be related to mothers of children with ASD. Older women with the support of a partner and with fewer children would seem more likely to achieve a more complex diagnosis requiring more assessments for their child than younger single mothers. Socio-demographic associations with ASD in most Western countries do not appear to operate as strongly and might even be absent in some Northern European countries. This might be due to a different social welfare structure in this region and specifically related to the universal screening for developmental disability. In addition to these and other social factors which could bias ascertainment, biological factors may be operating with older parents.

4. Immigrant status and ethnicity

Immigrant describes mothers who give birth while residing in a country which is not their own country of birth. *Ethnic* describes mothers who belong to a minority racial group in their country of residence which may or may not be their country of birth. To some extent, the groups of immigrant and ethnic mothers overlap. When examining social forces in relation to ASD and ID, it is important to take into account the often complex process associated with making a diagnosis of ASD.

4.1. Immigrant status

4.1.1. Immigrant mothers and autism

In all of the eight studies of immigrant mothers of children and ASD, [17, 22, 30, 57, 62, 75-77] the research concluded that immigrant mothers were more likely to have a child with ASD and particularly ASD with ID. [17, 22] In relation to immigrant mothers from Asia one of these studies was conducted by an Australian research group from New South Wales and used birth records and active surveillance to ascertain children with ASD. The group found that immigrant mothers born in South-East or North-East Asia were more likely to have a child with

ASD than other immigrant mothers. [57] A Western Australian study, using linked population data, also found that immigrant mothers from South-East or North-East Asia were at increased risk of having a child with ASD with ID. [17] A similar situation was described in Sweden where immigrant mothers from East Asia were more than three times as likely to have a child with ASD. [76]

Black immigrant mothers and immigrant mothers from developing countries were also found to be more likely to have a child with ASD compared to other immigrant mothers. One study from the UK [75] and another from Sweden [76] reported that black immigrant mothers [75] and immigrant mothers from sub-Saharan Africa [76] were much more likely to have a child with ASD compared to non-immigrant mothers. Further, a small Swedish case-control study compared the prevalence of autistic disorder and pervasive development disorder not otherwise specified (PDDNOS) in black African children with at least one parent born in Somali to the prevalence in children without a Somali background. [77] The researchers reported that these 17 black mothers were from three to four times more likely to have a child with ASD compared to the mothers without a Somali background. [77]

There is evidence that 'the intensity of the mother's skin colour' is related to her risk of having a child with ASD. A Swedish study compared the risk of ASD in the children of immigrants from each of North, East and other parts of Africa. [22] The mothers from North Africa were predominantly Moroccan and hence were probably fairer than the other two groups of mothers. For example, the East African group was predominantly from Somalia and Ethiopia while the ethnicity of the group from other parts of Africa was not described. The risk of ASD in the North African group was elevated (1.5) but not significantly higher than that of non-immigrant parents. On the other hand, the risk in the East African mothers and mothers from other parts of Africa of having a child with ASD was 1.9 and 3.5. [22]

Immigrant mothers from distant countries and those who emigrated during pregnancy were more likely to have a child with ASD than other immigrant mothers. For instance, researchers from the UK and Denmark found that immigrant mothers born outside of Europe were more likely to have a child with ASD. [62, 75] Similarly, a Swedish study found that immigrant mothers who were not from either of the US or Europe were nearly three times as likely to have a child with ASD compared to mothers from Nordic countries. [30] Another Swedish study ascertained that immigrant mothers who emigrated during pregnancy were even more likely to have a child with ASD than mothers who emigrated at other times. [22]

There is evidence that immigrant mothers are at different risks of ASD without ID and ASD with ID. Two Swedish studies found that immigrant mothers, excepting those from neighbouring Northern Europe, were less likely to have a child with ASD without ID [22] and Asperger syndrome [76] compared to non-immigrant mothers. One of these studies, along with an Australian study, reported that immigrant mothers were more likely to have a child with ASD with ID. [17, 22] In addition, the Swedish study found that the African immigrant mothers were more likely to have a child with ASD with ID compared to non-immigrant mothers. [22] Similar results were found in a small Swedish case-control study, where all seventeen of the Somali children with autism presented with ASD with ID. [77]

Another group of researchers reported that certain immigrant mothers were less likely to have a child with ASD than non-immigrant mothers. The US study conducted a national telephone survey which chose respondents who resided with their biological child and the child's other parent. [78] These researchers reported that non-immigrant Hispanic children had about twice the prevalence of ASD of immigrant Hispanic children. [78] These results were at variance to those in the previous studies of immigrant mothers. The lower likelihood of ASD in immigrant Hispanics compared to non-immigrant Hispanics could be explained by the relative ease of access of Mexican Hispanics to the US. With many countries, immigrants must meet stringent criteria prior to entry and some of these relate to the health of their offspring, their age, wealth, education and occupation. However, Mexican Hispanics would be less likely to experience the same stress, climatic change and exposure to new infections as most other immigrants groups. Moreover, immigrant parents from some of the other studies have usually relocated from more distant locations. For example, one reported findings which related to immigrants from Somali to Sweden, [77] another to non-European immigrants to Britain [75] and another to immigrants to the isolated continent of Australia. [57]

Overall, immigrant mothers and particularly black or Asian immigrant mothers, mothers from distant, developing countries and those who travelled while pregnant were at a higher risk of having a child with ASD. The mothers at highest risk of a child with ASD were from groups who would be expected to experience the most stress. For example, those relocating from a developing country and those pregnant at the time might be expected to experience higher stress than mothers who are relocating from a developed country or are not pregnant. This stress, along with the environmental changes associated with immigration, may have specific and negative effects on the developing fetal central nervous system. [22]

The risk of immigrant mothers having a child with ASD might be further exacerbated by an increased exposure to novel viruses [75] and intrauterine infections. [57] Other hypotheses to explain this association relate to low vitamin D levels [75, 79] and these have been further fuelled by animal studies. One study of rat pups with gross vitamin D deficiencies reported that they had structural brain abnormalities which were similar to those in children with ASD. [80] Furthermore, ASD was particularly common in black or Asian immigrant women and darker women more often have a vitamin D deficiency. [80] Generally, immigrant mothers are more likely to have a child with ASD with ID and less likely to have a child with ASD without ID. This may indicate different aetiologies for these subgroups.

Along with these biologically–based hypotheses, social factors may affect the likelihood of an immigrant mother having a child diagnosed with one of ASD, ASD with ID or ASD without ID. For instance, a diagnosis of ASD without ID would be particularly difficult where the child's parents were in an unfamiliar country, with a different language and where unusual behaviours might be explained by cultural differences. [22] In Australia, excluding the relatively small group of refugees, and in the US, Asian immigrants and their children are more often of a higher SES than other immigrant mothers. [81, 82] This might explain why the association with ASD was greater in this group than in other immigrant groups.

4.1.2. Immigrant mothers and intellectual disability

Compared to ASD, there was a reverse scenario identified with ID. Overall, immigrant mothers were 20-50% less likely to have a child with mild or moderate ID than non-immigrant mothers. [17, 20, 21] In Australia, Asian immigrant mothers were less likely to have a child with mild or moderate ID than non-immigrant mothers. [17, 20] As with ASD, the reversal with mild or moderate ID might be due to their higher SES compared to other immigrant groups. [81-83]

Differing results were found with the association of ID in the children of Mexican immigrants in a similar manner to the unexpected lower likelihood of Hispanic immigrant mothers having a child with ASD. A study of children with severe or profound ID, and born in California, found that immigrant mothers from Mexico, who would have been likely to be Hispanic, were nearly twice as likely to have a child with severe or profound ID compared to parents born in the US. [52] The idiosyncrasies associated with this immigrant group, compared to those immigrants from more distant locations, might explain this finding. They are likely to be less empowered than their non-immigrant counterparts and, as mentioned previously, their immigration was likely to be less regulated. Hence, from a socio-demographic viewpoint, they are more likely to present with low SES which is a risk factor for ID.

4.2. Ethnicity

In many studies, immigrant status and ethnicity were not differentiated. Therefore, within the ethnic group of mothers, there would have been mothers who, due to their country of birth, were both ethnic and immigrant. A recurrent trend of the research is that mothers from minority ethnic groups were less likely to have a child with ASD and more likely to have a child with ID than mothers who were not from minority ethnic groups.

Epidemiologists have found that mothers from ethnic minorities and particularly Aboriginal mothers were less likely to have a child with ASD. For example, in the US, the Hispanic mothers were less likely to have a child with ASD compared to non-Hispanic mothers. [23, 59, 84] In New York, the prevalence in Latinos was around half that in non-Latinos. [40] Some of these mothers from minority ethnic groups would have also been immigrant and, as reported, immigrant mothers usually have higher rates of ASD. This means that mothers from ethnic minority groups and who are native to their country might be expected to have the lowest likelihood of a child with ASD. This is the case in both Australia and Canada, where Aboriginal mothers had about half the odds of having a child with ASD compared to non-Aboriginal mothers [17, 29]

Compared to ASD, there was a reverse situation with ID since overall mothers from ethnic minority groups were more likely to have a child with ID. Asian mothers giving birth in California were 40% more likely to have a child with severe or profound ID although this result was not significant. [21] Hispanic mothers were more likely to have a child with either mild or moderate ID or severe or profound ID than Caucasian mothers. Again, in each of the ID groups, the results narrowly failed to achieve significance. [21] By comparison, Australian Aboriginal mothers were more than three times more likely to have a child with mild or moderate ID and were 60% more likely to have a child with severe or profound ID. [17, 20]

The higher rates of ID and the lower rates of ASD found in most ethnic minority and particularly indigenous communities may relate to the differing gene frequencies of these groups from the general population. However, differences could be exacerbated by environmental factors such as maternal alcohol consumption [85] without this being specifically identified as an aetiological factor. [86] Another consideration could be that marginalized groups are less empowered than others to pursue a diagnosis of ASD in contrast to a diagnosis of ID and that the infrastructures established for diagnostic assessment do not meet their needs. This second factor may also account for the lower prevalence of ASD and higher prevalence of ID with respect to the Australian Aboriginal community. [87]

In two Californian studies, contrasting findings were found for the previously described associations of ethnicity with ASD. Firstly, a cohort study found that Hispanic mothers were no less likely to have a child with ASD with ID than white mothers. [52] The same study also reported that Californian black mothers were more than five times as likely to have a child with ASD with ID as white mothers. [52] Furthermore, Californian Asian mothers were almost four times as likely to have a child with ASD with ID as white mothers. [52] Again, this may be a reflection of the higher proportion of immigrants in these groups. A second explanation in relation to the Asian mothers could be the fact that Asian mothers in US tend to have a higher SES than most other ethnic mothers. The second of the two Californian studies reported that Asian mothers giving birth in California were 30% less likely to have a child with mild or moderate ID. [21] This may also be a reflection of their higher SES.

4.3. Summary

Generally, immigrant mothers, and especially black and Asian immigrant mothers, were more likely to have a child with ASD compared to non-immigrant mothers. Furthermore, immigrant mothers were more likely to have a child with ASD with ID and less likely to have a child with ASD without ID compared to non-immigrant mothers. Immigrant mothers from distant or developing countries and mothers who emigrated when they were pregnant were even more likely to have a child with ASD. By contrast, in the US, Hispanic immigrant mothers were less likely to have a child with ASD than non-immigrant Hispanic mothers. Furthermore, non-immigrant mothers and particularly Aboriginal mothers were more likely to have a child with ID and especially mild or moderate ID than mothers who were not ethnic.

5. Health and associated characteristics

5.1. Mental health

The *World Health Organisation* describes mental health as a state of mental well-being. [88] This state of well-being can be enhanced by the prevention of mental disorders and the treatment and rehabilitation of those with mental disorders. Compromised mental health has been reported in the mothers of children with ASD and to a lesser extent in the mothers of children with ID compared to mothers of children without these disorders. For example, researchers found that mothers of a child with ASD were more likely to have a pre-existing psychiatric [62,

64, 89] or personality [62, 89, 90] disorder than mothers of typically developing children. Further, parents of a child with ASD were more likely to have increased rates of disorders which were related to affective disorder, [42] obsessive compulsive disorder, [27] anxiety, [27] paranoia, [27] and somatization [27] than the parents of typically developing children. One of these studies was conducted by a Californian team and recruited 269 parents of children with ASD via an existing university research program and control parents of typically developing children who were students (or their contacts) at the university. Self-reported mental health measures were obtained via questionnaire. [27] Other reported associations with parents of a child with ASD were increased rates of schizophrenia, [42, 89, 91] psychosis [42] and depression, [27, 64, 89] compared to the parents of typically developing children. Mothers of a child with ASD were more likely to have had pregnancies complicated by depression [92, 93] than mothers of typically developing children. Another research group explored mental health by comparing the rates of mental disorders in parents of people with ASD to those in parents of people with Down syndrome. [94] Parents of a child with ASD were more likely to have had an anxiety disorder than the parents of children with Down syndrome.

Studies have most commonly investigated the mental health of mothers of children with disabilities rather than the developmental outcomes in children born to mothers with mental health diagnoses. In one case-control study, the latter approach was employed and linked data from population-based registries was used to compare the likelihood of ASD with ID or ID in the children of more than 3 000 mothers with schizophrenia, bipolar disorder or unipolar major depression to the likelihood of these disorders in control mothers. Of these, around 1 300 mothers had bipolar disorder and these were assessed as nearly ten times more likely to have a child with ASD with ID than mothers without these disorders. [95] However, there were only four children with a mother with pre-existing bipolar disorder so these large odds are associated with particularly wide confidence intervals and only just reached significance.

The same study found that children of mothers with either schizophrenia, unipolar major depression or bipolar disorder or a combination of these disorders were about three times as likely to have a child with ID as mothers without these disorders. [95] Furthermore, mothers with ID themselves were more likely to have a child with ID compared to mothers with no history of psychiatric disorder or ID. [95]

5.2. Personality traits

Personality traits have been more often identified in the parents of children with ASD. For instance, parents of children with ASD were more likely to manifest a range of subtle autistic-like characteristics than parents of typically developing children. These characteristics have been grouped together as the Broad Autism Phenotype and include social cognition deficits, such as reasoning about the emotions of others, [96] autistic-like traits, [97] and impaired aspects of executive function. [98, 99]

A questionnaire entitled the Autism Spectrum Quotient (AQ) [100] was designed to assess the Broad Autism Phenotype in the five domains of social skills, communication, attention to detail, attention switching and imagination. [101] Researchers from the UK conducted a case-control study comprising parents of children with and without ASD from more than 1 500 families. Parents of children with ASD were more likely to exhibit autistic-like traits in all domains except that of attention to detail [102] than parents of typically developing children. Furthermore, these researchers and others found that a Broad Autism Phenotype occurred more commonly in parents of children with simplex ASD [97, 102] (where only one family member has ASD) and multiplex ASD [100, 103] (where more than one family member has ASD) than in parents of typically developing children. A dose-response effect was also described with parents in multiplex ASD families expressing a Broad Autism Phenotype significantly more often than parents in simplex ASD families. [32]

Some factors associated with maternal mental health may have a deleterious effect on the fetus and increase the likelihood of a child developing ASD or ID. For example, mothers with schizophrenia may remain on antipsychotic drugs during their pregnancies and these drugs, perhaps along with lower levels of maternal self-care (such as diet and medical care) and genetic factors related to the disease may adversely affect the development in the fetus. The milder autistic features in the parents of children with ASD might also be attributable to genetic factors associated with ASD. [33] In their affected children, these factors, along with additional genetic factors from the other parent, may sometimes produce the clinical phenotype of ASD.

5.3. Physical characteristics

Here are a group of diverse findings pertaining to the physical attributes of the mothers of interest. One study identified that mothers of children with ASD were significantly taller, particularly those of children with ASD without ID compared to the mothers of typically developing children. [17] This study population comprised more than 300 000 mothers and the mean heights of mothers of children with ASD with ID and mothers of children with ASD without ID were 164.3 and 164.9 cm. These means were significantly higher than the mean of the mothers of typically developing children (163.4cm). Another study found that mothers of children with ASD were both taller and heavier than mothers of typically developing children. [93] Similarly, a Canadian population study found that among non-smoking women, taller and heavier women were more likely to have a child with ASD compared to the mothers of typically developing children. [29]

Compared to the mothers of children with ASD, differing associations between maternal height and the mothers of children with ID were identified. Using population data, researchers identified that shorter women and those of medium height were more likely to have a child with mild or moderate ID than other mothers. [20] Further, the shortest group of women were more likely to have a child with severe or profound ID than other women. [20] Others found that mothers of children with mild or moderate ID, with a mean height of 162.1 cm were significantly shorter then than the mothers of typically developing children whose mean was 164.3 cm. However, the mothers of children with severe or profound ID were not significantly shorter than the mothers of typically developing children. [17] However, associations have also been described between SES and height, [104] and so the observed height differences between the mothers of children with ASD and ID may be a reflection of the different mean SES of these groups.

5.4. Health behaviours

Smoking during pregnancy has been associated with both ASD and ID in the offspring. In one study, mothers who smoked during pregnancy were reported to be more likely to have a child with ASD than mothers who did not smoke. [30] In 2011, a Swedish nested case-control study using medical registry data, found that mothers who smoked during early pregnancy were 70% less likely to have a child with ASD but almost twice as likely to have a child with Asperger syndrome. [76] This raises the possibility that Asperger syndrome has a distinct aetiology from other forms of ASD.

On the other hand, differing results were found in a US population-based, case-cohort study which explored the association of mothers who smoked during pregnancy and ASD. [105] Data from more than 6 000 000 mothers and their children were adjusted for potential confounders such as maternal age, education, and marital status. The definition of smoking during pregnancy was not described in the paper, so presumably this encompasses all mothers who had admitted to smoking one or more cigarettes during their pregnancy. The researchers reported that mothers who smoked during pregnancy were no more likely to have a child with ASD than mothers who did not smoke. Two large recently published cohort studies published in 2010 and 2011 also found no association between mothers who smoked during pregnancy and ASD. [29, 106] However, the first study examined only associations between maternal smoking and ASD generally [29] Hence, any associations between the relatively small group of mothers of children with Asperger syndrome may have been lost in the broader analysis. In addition, smoking was defined as *any smoking during pregnancy* which may have lessened the likelihood of an association with ASD. These were different outcomes to the second study, where mothers of children with ASD with ID and ASD without ID were considered separately and mothers who smoked ten or more cigarettes a day were a distinct group from the less intense smokers. [106] The first research group suggested that associations found with other studies were attributable to a confounding by maternal socio-demographic characteristics. [29]

The findings of associations between smoking during pregnancy and ID are also limited. A population study in the US ascertained that mothers who smoked 20 or more cigarettes a day were more likely to have a male child, but not a female child, with ID than mothers who did not smoke during pregnancy. [107] A large Finnish cohort study found that mothers who smoked after 2 months of pregnancy were no more likely to have a child with ID than mothers who did not smoke after this time. [46] This definition of smoking is broader than that of the first study so the likelihood of identifying an association between maternal smoking and ID may be reduced. Further, smoking during the first two months of pregnancy or gender of the fetus was not considered for inclusion in the model. An alternative study, with a more stringent definition of maternal smoking and which addressed these omissions, would be more likely to discern an association between smoking and ID.

Mothers who consume excessive alcohol during pregnancy were assessed as more likely to have a child with ID (but not ASD). This cause of ID is termed fetal alcohol syndrome (FAS) or fetal alcohol spectrum disorder (FASD). Fetal alcohol syndrome is at the most severe end of the spectrum and is diagnosed by characteristic facial features, brain dysmorphology, intellectual and other disabilities. [108] The milder diagnosis of FASD [109] does not require the presence of all of the characteristic physical features required for FAS. [110] Studies from Sweden and the US attributed between 2-10% of mild or moderate ID to FAS or FASD. [111, 112] While the US study considered that a further 3% of severe or profound ID was caused by FAS or FASD. [112]

In a Western Australian record linkage study heavy prenatal alcohol exposure was found to be an important cause, accounting for 2.5% of non-genetic intellectual disability. [85] Under-ascertainment, particularly of FASD, may result from non-disclosure of alcohol consumption during pregnancy due to the associated stigma. [113] In addition, perhaps due to inadequate training, [114] clinicians may lack awareness and confidence in making this diagnosis. [113] Also, clinicians may be concerned at the psychological effect on the mother of a FASD diagnosis and may not pursue this in situations where it is not conclusive or they feel it would not be beneficial to the mother or child.

Large cohort studies and linked data have provided researchers with the opportunity to study whole populations of mothers and their children with and without ASD and/or ID. Data can also be adjusted for a range of possible confounders such as SES and age. This enables the identification of new risk factors for ASD and/or ID and the elimination of others. For example, the association of smoking during pregnancy with ASD and/or ID in the offspring has weakened in the most recent studies using linked population data. Persisting associations are an increased risk of Asperger syndrome or PDD-NOS in mothers who smoked during pregnancy and an increased risk of ID in the male children of mothers who smoked heavily during pregnancy. Maternal alcohol consumption during pregnancy remains a risk factor for ID.

The remaining associations of maternal smoking with ASD and ID in the offspring could result from the effect of this exposure on overall fetal development and particularly growth restric-tion, [115, 116] preterm birth [115] and low birth-weight [117] Moreover, sub-optimal fetal growth has been associated with mild or moderate ID in Caucasian children. [118] The association of maternal alcohol consumption with ID might be due the multiple effects of alcohol on the fetus and placenta. [119] For example, alcohol can induce oxidative stress in placental villous tissue. Other demonstrated effects are an increase in neural tube defects and increased heart rate and cortisol levels in the exposed infant.

5.5. Physical health

The research literature has provided evidence that maternal physical health, both prior to and during pregnancy is related to the likelihood of a mother having a child with ASD and/or ID. Various pre-existing conditions in the mother and related or unrelated complications of her pregnancy increase the likelihood of a mother having a child with ASD and/or ID compared to mothers who do not have the condition.

Pre-pregnancy obesity is an example of a condition which increases the likelihood of a woman having a child with ASD and/or ID. Obese women were more likely to have a child with ASD, [24, 54, 120] or ID [24, 46] than women who were not obese. One of these studies was a Finnish study which used linked data from the birth cohorts of 1966 and

1985-6 and included around 250 mothers of children with ID in each of the cohorts. [46]
In both cohorts, mothers with obesity prior to their pregnancies were more likely to have
a child with ID than women without pre-pregnancy obesity. However, the association of
ID with pre-pregnancy obesity was an increasing risk reflected in the greater odds in the
latter cohort(2.4) compared with the original cohort(1.8). [46] Another of the research
groups reported that women with an early age of menarche were more likely to have a
child with ASD than other women. [120] Early menarche, along with pre-pregnancy
obesity, could indicate the possibility of maternal hormonal involvement in the risk of ASD
and ID. [120] Then again, the relationship with ID may be resulting from confounding by
the association between socioeconomic disadvantage and obesity in highly developed
countries. [121] In the light of the increasing prevalence of obesity in these countries, these
associations with ASD and ID are an important future research direction. [122]

Women with an auto-immune disorder or anomalies of the immune system were more likely
to have a child with ASD and/or ID than women who did not. [25, 26, 123] Furthermore, the
majority of associations in this area were with ASD rather than ID. For example, in a case-
control study using linked data with more than 1 200 cases, mothers with an auto-immune
disorder were 60% more likely to have a child with ASD than mothers without an auto-immune
disorder. [26] These findings were supported by a small case-control study of 61 mothers of
children with ASD. [123] Other studies have found that women with a particular auto-immune
disease were more likely to have a child with ASD than women who did not have the disease.
For instance, a case-control study with 407 cases found that women with psoriasis were more
likely to have a child with ASD than mothers without this disorder. [124] Another research
group used linked population data with more than 3 000 mothers of a child with ASD and
nearly 700 000 control mothers. They reported that women with rheumatoid arthritis or celiac
disease were more likely to have a child with ASD than mothers who did not have one of these
disorders. [125]

One study found that women with pre-existing diabetes were more likely to have a child
with ASD than women without pre-existing diabetes [29] However, a study used linked
data from the national birth and inpatient registries and reported that women with pre-
existing diabetes were no more likely to have a child with ASD than other mothers. [30]
In relation to ID, a group of US researchers investigated a possible association with diabetes
by comparing more than 160 000 mother-child dyads. The researchers identified that
mothers with pre-existing diabetes were more than 10% more likely to have a child with
ID. [126] Diabetes during pregnancy was also associated with both ASD and ID. For
instance, two studies found that mothers with diabetes during pregnancy were more likely
to have a child with ASD [25] and ASD with ID [127] than mothers without the disorder. The first of these was a Canadian population study which included nearly 800 cases
of ASD and more than 66 000 births. Mothers who developed gestational diabetes were
associated with a 76% increased risk of ASD compared to women who did not develop
the condition. [25] The second was an Australian population study which found that
mothers who had diabetes during pregnancy were nearly three times as likely to have a
child with ASD with ID than mothers without diabetes. [127] More attenuated results were

ascertained by Californian researchers who conducted a case-control study and compared the mothers of more than 500 children with ASD, 172 mothers of children with developmental disabilities other than ASD to typically developing children. [24] They found that mothers with gestational diabetes were more likely (but not significantly more likely) to have a child with ASD than mothers without the disorder. The lack of significance may be due to the reduced power of this smaller study. Two studies identified an association between gestational diabetes and ID or a condition similar to ID. [24, 127] One was a large retrospective cohort study using linked registry data. Here the researchers found that mothers with diabetes during pregnancy were nearly 70% more likely to have a child with mild or moderate ID [127] compared to mothers without this disorder. The other research group found that mothers with diabetes during pregnancy were nearly two and a half times more likely to have a child with a developmental disability other than ASD than mothers without diabetes during pregnancy. [24]

Further, differences have been identified relating to the immunological status of mothers of children with ASD prior to their pregnancies. An independent case-control study identified fetal brain antibodies in mothers of children with ASD but not in controls mothers. [128] This study found that mothers of children with ASD were significantly more likely to have an auto-antibody reactivity pattern for human fetal brain proteins than mothers of typically developing children.

Cytokines are regulators of immune response and maternal immune dysfunction has been associated with the neurological development of the fetus. [129] A case-control study identified that mothers of children with ASD and/or ID were more likely to have aberrant cytokine profiles compared to the mothers of typically developing children. [130] In this study, the concentration of serum cytokines at mid-pregnancy in the mothers of children with ASD with ID, developmental disabilities other than ASD and typically developing children were compared. Mothers of a child with ASD with ID were more likely to have higher concentrations of three particular cytokines than mothers of a typically developing child. In addition, mothers of a child with a developmental disability other than ASD were more likely to have higher concentrations of a different set of three different cytokines (to the ASD group) than mothers of typically developing children. [130]

Auto-immune diseases and other immune dysfunction might impinge on the immature nervous system of the developing fetus. This could have a deleterious effect on future cognitive function [131] and increase the likelihood of ASD and ID. [130]

Hypertension or high blood pressure is either a temporary or sustained elevation of the blood pressure in the arteries. [132] Moreover, the elevation is at a level where cardiovascular or other damage may occur. Hypertension during pregnancy was associated with an increased risk of ASD in the child. Three studies provided evidence that women who experienced hypertension during pregnancy were more likely to have a child with ASD [24, 30, 54] than women who had not suffered hypertension. In one of the studies, Swedish researchers conducted a nested, matched case-control study with data from over 400 children with ASD and over 2 000 controls. [30] Records of children's hospitalisation over 10 years were linked to birth records. The researchers concluded that mothers who suffered a hypertensive disease during pregnancy were 60% more likely to have a child with ASD than other mothers. In contrast, a large cohort study of more than 650 000 nurses found that mothers with hypertension during pregnancy were no more likely to have a child with ASD than mothers without with hypertension during pregnancy. [25] Possibly, these nurses, with their increased medical knowledge, sought treatment before their blood pressure reached a level which would have been damaging to the unborn child.

Hypertension and oedema are two common symptoms of pre-eclampsia or toxaemia [132] which is a condition occurring in about 8% of first pregnancies. [133] Women who experience this condition, along with those who suffer oedema, were more likely to have a child with ASD and/or ID. Three groups of researchers found that women with pre-eclampsia [25, 29, 134] and those suffering oedema [92] during their pregnancies were more likely to have a child with ASD than women without these conditions during their pregnancies. In contrast, a much smaller case-control study, found that woman with pre-eclampsia had reduced (though not significantly so) likelihood of a child with ASD. [60] Pre-eclampsia was also associated with ID. [135] This association was found by researchers in a population-based, retrospective cohort study in South Carolina. Here, women who suffered pre-eclampsia were nearly 60% more likely to have a child with ID.

Associations of maternal epilepsy have been demonstrated with both ASD and ID. Women who experienced epilepsy during pregnancy were more likely to have a child with ASD with ID [127] or mild or moderate ID. [127] These Australian researchers conducted a retrospective cohort study of nearly 3 000 mothers of children with ASD and/or ID of unknown cause and around 237 000 mothers of typically developing children using linked population data from medical registries. They established that mothers with epilepsy during pregnancy were more than four and a half times as likely to have a child with ASD with ID [127] and more than three and a half times as likely to have a child with mild or moderate ID compared to mothers without epilepsy during their pregnancies. [127] A case-control study in US had only 61 control mothers of a child with ASD. [123] Here, mothers who had experienced seizure prior to their pregnancies were nearly six times as likely to have a child with ASD. However, possibly due to the small size of the study, results did not reach significance.

In addition to epilepsy, mothers who experienced a range of other conditions during pregnancy were found to be more likely to have a child with ASD than other mothers. Overall, health issues during pregnancy were associated with a higher risk of ASD. Researchers reported that women who had allergies, [124] asthma, [124] bleeding, [30] or high body temperature [93] during their pregnancies were more likely to have a child with ASD than women who had not experienced these conditions during their pregnancies. Asthma during pregnancy was also associated with ID, with pregnant women with asthma being more likely to have a child with mild or moderate ID than mothers without this condition during pregnancy. [127]

Other conditions during pregnancy have been associated with ID. For instance, an Australian population study found that women who had renal or urinary conditions during pregnancy were more than twice as likely to have a child with mild or moderate ID as women without these conditions during pregnancy. [127] Furthermore, women who suffered anaemia during their pregnancies were more than five times as likely to have a child with severe or profound ID than women without anaemia during pregnancy. [127] Two research groups ascertained that infections during pregnancy were associated with ASD. They found that women whose pregnancies were complicated by urinary tract infection, [93] or any bacterial or viral infection [93, 136] were more likely to have a child with ASD than mothers who did not experience an infection.

Infections during pregnancy were also associated with ID. For example, one study reported that mothers who suffered trichomoniasis during pregnancy were more likely to have a child with ID than mothers without this condition during pregnancy. [137] A cohort study used Medicaid claims and linked infant records to investigate the association of treated and untreated urinary tract infections during pregnancy with later ID in the child. [138] The researchers reported that pregnant women with untreated urinary tract infections were 30% more likely to have a child with ID than pregnant women without these infections. Moreover, mothers with untreated urinary tract infections were 22% more likely to have a child with ID than mothers with antibiotic treated urinary tract infections. [138]

There is always a risk that the use of certain medications during pregnancy may have adverse effects on a developing fetus. This use is likely to be related to a woman's health and the decision to use a particular medication at this time must be difficult. Sometimes, medications initially considered safe have been later implicated to adversely affect the future health of the unborn child. For instance, six studies found that the children of mothers who used anti-depressants, [64, 139] anti-convulsants, [140] psycho-active drugs, [64] prescribed medications [54, 93] and medications generally [141] had a higher risk of a child with ASD. One of these was a population-based case-control study in Stockholm. [64] Using registry data, the researchers assessed that mothers who took psycho-active drugs or anti-depressants during their pregnancies were more than four times as likely to have a child with ASD.

It is also possible that the increased use of prescribed medications in mothers of children with ASD may have resulted from a bias in data collection. In one of the studies which found an increased use of prescribed medications, case mothers were recruited via their response to an advertisement in a support agency newsletter or via their membership of a support agency. [93] Each of these methods might have resulted in a bias in the direction of a high SES. This, in turn, may have produced an increased use of prescribed medications in the case mothers. On the other hand, the study which found an increased use of medications generally was a population study using medical registries. [141] The reported associations are likely to be mediated by a complex interaction of factors. For instance, in addition to possible SES bias, there could be a genetic association such as the familial link of depressive disorders or epilepsy with ASD. Another possibility is an environmental effect which results from the physiological impact of maternal medication use on the uterine environment.

5.6. Summary

Before the birth of their affected children, certain socio-demographic, health and physical attributes differentiate mothers of children with ASD and/or ID from those of mothers in the general population. Further, these attributes often vary by the disability group of their child. In Tables 2 to 4, these differences are grouped into categories according to their associations with groups of mothers. An examination of Table 2 shows that with socio-demographic factors, the relationships with ASD and ID are most often reversed. High SES was most often associated with the ASD groups of mothers and low SES, most often associated with ID.

Different associations of marital status were found with each of ASD and ID. With ASD, the only two studies found in the area had opposing results. With all but one study, single mothers were at increased risk of unspecified ID and mild or moderate ID, compared to women who were living with a partner.

In the majority of the studies, increased maternal age, along with increased paternal and parental age, were associated with ASD and ASD without ID. With ID, two associations emerged. Younger mothers had an increased risk of bearing a child with mild or moderate ID. But severe or profound ID was associated with increased maternal age.

Lower parity had a consistent positive association with ASD in most studies. With mild or moderate ID and unspecified ID, the relationship was reversed and the association was with greater parity. However, with severe or profound ID, there was no association.

In Table 3, the associations with immigrant status and ethnicity are summarized. Most often, immigrant mothers are more likely to have a child with ASD or ASD with ID than non-immigrant mothers. On the other hand, ASD without ID was associated with non-immigrants, excepting those immigrants from nearby countries. The Mexican/Hispanic immigrant mothers in the US were a separate group since these mothers were less likely to have a child with ASD than Mexican/Hispanic non-immigrant mothers.

With ethnicity, the associations differed from those with immigrant status, in spite of the overlap between the groups. Except for Asian and black mothers, mothers from ethnic minority groups were at a lower risk of children with ASD compared to Caucasian mothers. With the exception of Asian mothers, the relationship with ID was reversed since mothers from ethnic minority groups, and particularly Aboriginal mothers, were at an increased risk of a child with ID.

Table 4 shows the many associations of health and behavioural traits with ASD and highlights the quite small proportion common to both ASD and ID. With mental health, ten research groups reported associations with ASD. Contrastingly, only one study found an association with the mothers of children with ID. Autistic-like traits were associated only with the parents of children with ASD.

As with other socio-demographic factors, ASD and ID had an overall reverse association with height. Taller and heavier women were more likely to have offspring with ASD and shorter women to have offspring with ID. The associations with maternal smoking during pregnancy were minimal. Excessive alcohol consumption during pregnancy was only associated with offspring with ID. Obesity though was associated with both ASD and ID.

Both ASD and ID had associations with immune function, though the association with ASD was broader. Both pre-existing diabetes and diabetes during pregnancy were associated with ASD and/or ID. Further, abnormal levels of cytokines during pregnancy were also associated with each of ASD and ID. Other associations were with only ASD and were auto-immune disorder generally, psoriasis, rheumatoid arthritis, celiac disease and maternal fetal brain antibodies.

Seven studies associated hypertension, oedema and pre-eclampsia with ASD whereas only one study associated pre-eclampsia with ID. Epilepsy and asthma had associations with both of ASD and ID but no other associations during pregnancy were common to both disorders. Medication use during pregnancy was only found to be associated with ASD.

	ASD			ID		
Category	ASD without ID	Undifferentiated ASD	ASD with ID	Mild ID	Unspecified ID	Severe ID
SES	+veassoc [17,47]	+veassoc [17,39-41,47]	+veassoc [17]	-veassoc [17,20,48]	-veassoc [21,44-46,48]	
In Denmark & Sweden		No assoc[42] -veassoc[43]				
Education as a measure of SES	+veassoc [47]	+veassoc [21,41,50]		-veassoc [20,21]	-veassoc [20,21,32,44,45,51,53] -veassoc (DD)[24]	-veassoc [21,52]
Marital status at child's birth (Women with partners)		+veassoc [17] -veassoc [54]	+veassoc [17]	-veassoc [20]	-veassoc[17] -veassoc (early cognitive delay) [55]	
Age Maternal	+veassoc [17,47]	+veassoc [17,21,29,47,56-61]		-veassoc [17,20,21]	No assoc [46]	+veassoc [21,68]
Paternal & maternal		+veassoc [17,56,58,61]				
Only paternal	+veassoc [65]	+veassoc [58,62-65]				
Maternal & paternal (Denmark, Sweden & UK)		No assoc [42,43,66]				
Lower parity	+veassoc [17,74]	+veassoc [29,41,73] -veassoc [25] No assoc [42]	+veassoc [17]	-veassoc [17,20,21]	-veassoc [21,46]	No assoc [21,52]
Age & lower parity		+veassoc [58]				

ASD, autism spectrum disorder; ID, intellectual disability; Mild ID, Mild or moderate ID; Severe ID, Severe or profound ID; SES, socio-economic status; +ve, positive; -ve, negative; assoc, association.

Table 2. Associations of socio-demographic factors in the mothers of children with ASD and/or ID

		ASD		ID	
Category	ASD without ID	Undifferentiated ASD	ASD with ID	Mild ID	Severe ID
Immigrant status (Immigrant vs non-immigrant)		+veassoc[17,22,30,57,62,75-77]	+veassoc [17,22]	-veassoc[17,20,21]	
North Europe & UK	-veassoc (except other North Europeans)[22,76]		+veassoc in Somalis[77] & Africans [22]		
US		-veassoc immigrant Hispanic vs non-immigrant Hispanics [78]			+veassoc Mexican immigrants in California [52]
Asian		+veassoc in SE & NE Asians [17,57]+veassoc in East Asians[76]		-veassoc for Asians in Aus& US [17,20]	
Ethnicity(Non-Caucasian vs Caucasians)		-veassoc in Hispanics [23,59,84] & Latinos [40]		+veassoc in Aboriginals [17,20]	+veassoc in Aboriginals [17,20]
		-veassoc in Aboriginals [17,29]			
		+veassoc in Asians [52] +veassoc in Blacks [52]	No assoc in Hispanics [52]	-veassoc in Asians [21]	

ASD, autism spectrum disorder; ID, intellectual disability; Mild ID, Mild or moderate ID; Severe ID, Severe or profound ID; +ve, positive; -ve, negative;assoc, association; SE, south eastern; NE, north eastern; Aus, Australia; NHW, non-Hispanic white.

Table 3. Associations of immigrant status and ethnicity in the mothers of children with ASD and/or ID

	ASD		ID
Category	ASD without ID, [Asperger syndrome] [ASD with ID]	Undifferentiated ASD	Unspecified ID[Mild ID], [Severe ID]
Mental health		Schizophrenia [42,89,91]	Schizophrenia [95] or
		Depression [27,64,89]	Unipolar major depression [95] or
	Bipolar disorder [ASD with ID] [95]		Bipolar disorder [95]
		Psychiatric, [62,64,89] personality disorders, [62,89,90] affective [42] & obsessive compulsive disorders,[27] anxiety, [27,94] & paranoia [27]Somatization, [27] psychosis,[42] depression,[27, 64, 89] & depression during pregnancy [92,93]	ID in mother [95]
Personality traits		Autistic-like traits [97,100,102,103]	
Physical characteristics	Taller[ASD without ID] [17 [17]Taller[ASD with ID] [17]	Taller and heavier [93] Taller and heavier (non-smoking mothers only) [29]	Shorter, medium height [20]Shortest[Severe ID] [20] & shorter[Mild ID] [17]
Health behaviours During pregnancy	Smoking[Asperger syndrome] [76]	Smoking [30]Smoking(-veassoc) [76] Smoking(no assoc) [29,105,106]	In male children with ≥ 20 cigs/day in mother[107]Smoking (no assoc)[46]
			Alcohol[85]Alcohol[Mild ID] [111, 112] Alcohol[Severe ID] [112]
Physical health	Obesity[ASD with ID] [24]	Obesity [24,54,120]	Obesity [24,46]
		Early menarche[120]	
Immune function	Diabetes during pregnancy [ASD with ID] [127]	Diabetes[24,29] & diabetes during pregnancy[25]	Diabetes[126] & diabetes during pregnancy(Mild ID)[127] & (DD no ASD)[24]
		Higher conc of 3 cytokines[130]	Higher conc of 3 other cytokines(DD) [130]
		Any auto-immune disorder, [256,26,123] psoriasis,[124] & rheumatoid arthritis[125] celiac disease, [125] &fetal brain antibodies [128]	

ASD, autism spectrum disorder; ID, intellectual disability; Mild ID, mild or moderate ID; Severe ID, severe or profound ID; UTI, urinary tract infection,

Table 4. Associations of mental health, personality traits, physical characteristics, health behaviours and physical health in the mothers of children with ASD and/or ID

	ASD		ID
Category	ASD without ID[ASD with ID]	**Undifferentiated ASD**	**Unspecified ID[Mild ID], [Severe ID]**
Other areas during pregnancy		Hypertension[24,30,54] Oedema[92]	
		Pre-eclampsia[25,29,134]	Pre-eclampsia[135]
	Epilepsy[ASD with ID] [127]		Epilepsy(Mild ID)[127]
		Allergies,[124] bleeding,[30] & high temperature[93] UTI[93] & any infection[93,136]	Renal/urinary conditions,[127] [Mild ID][126] Anaemia [Severe ID] [127]Trichomoniasis[137] & untreated UTI[138]
		Asthma [124]	Asthma (Mild ID) [127]
		Anti-depressants,[64,139] prescribed[54,93] & other medications[141] Anticonvulsants[140] & psycho-active drugs[64]	

ASD, autism spectrum disorder; ID, intellectual disability; Mild ID, mild or moderate ID; Severe ID, severe or profound ID; UTI, urinary tract infection.

Table 5. Associations of health during pregnancy in the mothers of children with ASD and/or ID

6. Conclusion

This chapter provides a review of the research pertaining to the pre-existing characteristics of mothers of a child with ASD and/or ID. Some consistent and enduring associations have emerged across the published reports. With socio-demographic factors, these are the contrasting associations of maternal education, age, immigrant status and ethnicity with ASD and ID. With maternal health; aspects of mental health, personality traits, immune function and the use of medication during pregnancy have stronger associations with the mothers of children with ASD than ID. Some of these differences may be reflections of distinct aetiologies for ASD and/or ID of unknown cause and provide directions for future research. As such, primary and secondary prevention strategies may be refined and/or developed which will contribute to lower prevalence, reduced levels of severity and better outcomes for affected children.

Author details

Jenny Fairthorne*, Amanda Langridge, Jenny Bourke and Helen Leonard*

*Address all correspondence to: jfairthorne@ichr.uwa.edu.au

Centre for Child Health, University of Western Australia, Australia

References

[1] Filipek, P., et al., The screening and diagnosis of autistic spectrum disorders. Journal of Autism and Developmental Disorders, 1999. 29(6): p. 439-84.

[2] American Psychiatric Association, Diagnostic and Statistical Manual of Mental Disorders, Fourth Edition, 2000, American Psychiatric Association: Washington, DC.

[3] Rutter, M., Aetiology of autism: findings and questions. Journal of Intellectual Disability Research, 2005. 49(4): p. 231-38.

[4] Robinson, P., et al., Genetically determined low maternal serum dopamine hydroxylase levels and the etiology of autism spectrum disorders. American Journal of Medical Genetics, 2001. 100(1): p. 30-6.

[5] Trajkovski, V., Etiology of autism. Journal of Special Education, 2004. 5(1-2): p. 61-74.

[6] Bass, M., et al., Genetic studies in autistic disorder and chromosome 15. Neurogenetics, 2000. 2(4): p. 219-26.

[7] Brune, C., et al., 5-HTTLPR genotype-specific phenotype in children and adolescents with autism. American Journal of Psychiatry, 2006. 163(12): p. 2148-56.

[8] Newschaffer, C., et al., The epidemiology of autism spectrum disorders. Annual Review of Public Health, 2007. 28(21): p. 235-58.

[9] Mefford, H., M. Batshaw, and E. Hoffman, Genomics, intellectual disability, and autism. New England Journal of Medicine, 2012. 366(8): p. 733-43.

[10] Stoltenberg, C., et al., The autism birth cohort (ABC): a paradigm for gene-environment-timing research. Molecular Psychiatry, 2011. 15(7): p. 676-80.

[11] Kubota, T., et al., Novel etiological and therapeutic strategies for neurodiseases: epigenetic understanding of gene-environment interactions. Journal of Pharmacological Sciences, 2010. 113: p. 3-8.

[12] Dodge, K. and M. Rutter, Gene-environment interactions: state of the science, in Gene-environment interactions in developmental psychopathology, K. Dodge and M. Rutter, Editors. 2011, Guilford Press: New York.

[13] Maher, P., Methylglyoxal, advanced glycation end products and autism: Is there a connection? Medical Hypotheses, 2012.

[14] Young, D., et al., The diagnosis of autism in a female: Could it be Rett syndrome? European Journal of Pediatrics, 2008. 167(6): p. 661-9.

[15] Oberlé, I., et al., Instability of a 550-base pair DNA segment and abnormal methylation in Fragile X syndrome. Science, 1991. 252(5009): p. 1097-102.

[16] Fombonne, E., Epidemiology of pervasive developmental disorders. Pediatric Research, 2009. 65(6): p. 591-8.

[17] Leonard, H., et al., Autism and intellectual disability are differentially related to sociodemographic background at birth. PLoS ONE, 2011. 6(3): p. e17875.

[18] Matson, J. and M. Shoemaker, Intellectual disability and its relationship to autism spectrum disorders. Research in Developmental Disabilities, 2009. 30(6): p. 1107-14.

[19] Leonard, H. and X. Wen, The epidemiology of mental retardation: challenges and opportunities in the new millennium. Mental Retardation and Developmental Disabilities Research Reviews, 2002. 8(3): p. 117-34.

[20] Leonard, H., et al., Association of sociodemographic characteristics of children with intellectual disability in Western Australia. Social Science and Medicine, 2005. 60(7): p. 1499-513.

[21] Croen, L., J. Grether, and S. Selvin, The epidemiology of mental retardation of unknown cause. Pediatrics, 2001. 107(6): p. e86.

[22] Magnusson, C., et al., Migration and autism spectrum disorder: population-based study. British Journal of Psychiatry, 2012.

[23] Pinborough-Zimmerman, J., et al., Sociodemographic risk factors associated with autism spectrum disorders and intellectual disability. Autism Research, 2011. 4(5).

[24] Krakowiak, P., et al., Maternal metabolic conditions and risk for autism and other neurodevelopmental disorders. Pediatrics, 2012. 129(5).

[25] Lyall, K., et al., Pregnancy complications and obstetric suboptimality in association with autism spectrum disorders in children of the Nurses' Health Study II. Autism Research, 2012. 5(1): p. 21-30.

[26] Keil, A., et al., Parental autoimmune diseases associated with autism spectrum disorders in offspring. Epidemiology, 2010. 21(6): p. 805-8.

[27] Hodge, D., C. Hoffman, and D. Sweeney, Increased psychopathology in parents of children with autism: genetic liability or burden of caregiving? Journal of Developmental and Physical Disabilities, 2011. 23(3): p. 227-39.

[28] Morgan, V., et al., What impact do obstetric complications have on the risk of ad-verse psychiatric outcomes for the high risk children of mothers with schizophrenia and other psychoses? Schizophrenia Research, 2008. 102(Supplement 2): p. 167-8.

[29] Burstyn, I., F. Sithole, and L. Zwaigenbaum, Autism spectrum disorders, maternal characteristics and obstetric complications among singletons born in Alberta, Cana-da. Chronic Diseases in Canada, 2010. 30(4): p. 125-34.

[30] Hultman, C., P. Sparen, and S. Cnattingius, Perinatal risk factors for infantile autism. Epidemiology, 2002. 13(4): p. 417-23.

[31] Losh, M., et al., Neuropsychological profile of autism and the broad autism pheno-type. Archives of General Psychiatry, 2009. 66(5): p. 518-26.

[32] Losh, M., et al., Defining key features of the broad autism phenotype: a comparison across parents of multiple and single incidence autism families. American Journal of Medical Genetics, 2008. 147(4): p. 424-33.

[33] Piven, J., The broad autism phenotype: a complementary strategy for molecular ge-netic studies of autism. American Journal of Medical Genetics, 2001. 105(1): p. 34-5.

[34] Harvey, J., M. O'Callaghan, and B. Vines, Prevalence of maternal depression and its relationship to ADL skills in children with developmental delay. Journal of Paediat-rics and Child Health, 1997. 33(1): p. 42-6.

[35] Hertz-Picciotto, I., et al., The CHARGE Study: an epidemiologic investigation of ge-netic and environmental factors contributing to autism. Environmental Health Per-spectives, 2006. 114(7): p. 1119-25.

[36] Spitzer, R. and B. Siegel, The DSM-III-R field trial of pervasive developmental disor-ders. Journal of the American Academy of Child and Adolescent Psychiatry, 1990. 29(6): p. 855-62.

[37] Western Australian Autism Diagnosticians' Forum. Diagnosis in Western Australia 2012; Available from: http://waadf.org.au/Waitlist_times_1_December_2011.pdf.

[38] Shattuck, P. and S. Grosse, Issues related to the diagnosis and treatment of autism spectrum disorders. Mental Retardation and Developmental Disabilities Research Reviews, 2007. 13(2): p. 129-35.

[39] Durkin, M., et al., Socioeconomic inequality in the prevalence of autism spectrum disorder: evidence from a US cross-sectional study. PLoS ONE, 2010. 5(7): p. e11551.

[40] Liptak, G., et al., Disparities in diagnosis and access to health services for children with autism: data from the National Survey of Children's Health. Journal of Develop-mental and Behavioral Pediatrics, 2008. 29(3): p. 152-60.

[41] King, M. and P. Bearman, Socioeconomic status and the increased prevalence of au-tism in California. American Sociological Review, 2011. 76(2): p. 320-46.

[42] Larsson, H., et al., Risk factors for autism: perinatal factors, parental psychiatric his-
      tory, and socioeconomic status. American Journal of Epidemiology, 2005. 161(10): p.
      916-25.

[43] Rai, D., et al., Parental socioeconomic status and risk of offspring autism spectrum
      disorders in a Swedish population-based study. Journal of the American Academy of
      Child and Adolescent Psychiatry, 2012.

[44] Gissler, M., et al., Social class differences in health until the age of seven years among
      the Finnish 1987 birth cohort. Social Science and Medicine, 1998. 46(12): p. 1543-52.

[45] Zheng, X., et al., Socioeconomic status and children with intellectual disability in
      China. Journal of Intellectual Disability Research, 2012. 56(2): p. 212-20.

[46] Heikura, U., et al., Variations in prenatal sociodemographic factors associated with
      intellectual disability: a study of the 20-year interval between two birth cohorts in
      Northern Finland. American Journal of Epidemiology, 2008. 167(2): p. 169-77.

[47] Bhasin, T. and D. Schendel, Sociodemographic risk factors for autism in a US metro-
      politan area. Journal of Autism and Developmental Disorders, 2007. 37(4): p. 667-77.

[48] Emerson, E., Deprivation, ethnicity and the prevalence of intellectual and develop-
      mental disabilities. Journal of Epidemiology and Community Health, 2012. 66(3): p.
      218-24.

[49] Harris, J., Autism risk factors: moving from epidemiology to translational epidemiol-
      ogy. Journal of the American Academy of Child and Adolescent Psychiatry, 2012.
      51(5).

[50] Van Meter, K., et al., Geographic distribution of autism in California: a retrospective
      birth cohort analysis. Autism Research, 2010. 3(1): p. 19-29.

[51] Yaqoob, M., et al., Mild intellectual disability in children in Lahore, Pakistan: aetiolo-
      gy and risk factors. Journal of Intellectual Disability Research, 2004. 48(7): p. 663-71.

[52] Jelliffe-Pawlowski, L., et al., Risks for severe mental retardation occurring in isolation
      and with other developmental disabilities. American Journal of Medical Genetics,
      2005. 136(2): p. 152-7.

[53] Singhi, P., et al., Psychosocial problems in families of disabled children. British Jour-
      nal of Medical Psychology, 1990. 63(2): p. 173-82.

[54] Dodds, L., et al., The role of prenatal, obstetric and neonatal factors in the develop-
      ment of autism. Journal of Autism and Developmental Disorders, 2011. 41(7): p.
      891-902.

[55] Hatton, E., et al., Changes in family composition and marital status in families with a
      young child with cognitive delay. Journal of Applied Research in Intellectual Disabil-
      ities, 2010. 23(1): p. 14-26.

[56] King, M., et al., Estimated autism risk and older reproductive age. American Journal of Public Health, 2009. 99(9): p. 1673-9.

[57] Williams, K., et al., Perinatal and maternal risk factors for autism spectrum disorders in New South Wales, Australia. Child-care, Health and Development, 2008. 34(2): p. 249-56.

[58] Durkin, M., et al., Advanced parental age and the risk of autism spectrum disorder. American Journal of Epidemiology, 2008. 168(11): p. 1268-76.

[59] Windham, G., et al., Birth prevalence of autism spectrum disorders in the San Francisco Bay area by demographic and ascertainment source characteristics. Journal of Autism and Developmental Disorders, 2011. 41(10): p. 1362-72.

[60] Stein, D., et al., Obstetric complications in individuals diagnosed with autism and in healthy controls. Comprehensive Psychiatry, 2006. 47(1): p. 69-75.

[61] El-Baz , F., et al., Risk factors for autism: an Egyptian study. Egyptian Journal of Medical Human Genetics, 2011. 12: p. 31-8.

[62] Lauritsen, M., C. Pedersen, and P. Mortensen, Effects of familial risk factors and place of birth on the risk of autism: a nationwide register-based study. Journal of Child Psychology and Psychiatry, 2005. 46(9): p. 963-71.

[63] Reichenberg, A., R. Gross, and M. Weiser, Advancing paternal age and autism. Archives of General Psychiatry, 2006. 63(9): p. 1026-32.

[64] Eriksson, M., et al., First-degree relatives of young children with autism spectrum disorders: some gender aspects. Research in Developmental Disabilities, 2012. 33(5): p. 1642-8.

[65] Tsuchiya, K., et al., Paternal age at birth and high-functioning autistic-spectrum disorder in offspring. British Journal of Psychiatry, 2008. 193(4): p. 316-21.

[66] Robinson, E., et al., Brief report: no association between parental age and extreme social-communicative autistic traits in the general population. Journal of Autism and Developmental Disorders, 2011. 41(12): p. 1733-7.

[67] Frenette, P., et al., Factors affecting the age at diagnosis of autism spectrum disorders in Nova Scotia, Canada. Autism, 2011: p. 1-12.

[68] Drews, C., et al., Variation in the influence of selected sociodemographic risk factors for mental retardation. American Journal of Public Health, 1995. 85(3): p. 329-34.

[69] Hook, E. and A. Lindsjö, Down syndrome in live births by single year maternal age interval in a Swedish study: comparison with results from a New York State study. American Journal of Human Genetics, 1978. 30(1): p. 19-27.

[70] Liu, K., N. Zerubavel, and P. Bearman, Social demographic change and autism. Demography, 2010. 47(2): p. 327-43.

[71] Hultman, C., et al., Advancing paternal age and risk of autism: new evidence from a population-based study and a meta-analysis of epidemiological studies. Molecular Psychiatry, 2011. 16(12): p. 1203-12.

[72] Mosby's Medical Dictionary 2009: Elsevier. 8th edition.

[73] Glasson, E., et al., Perinatal factors and the development of autism: a population study. Archives of General Psychiatry, 2004. 61(6): p. 618-27.

[74] Schmidt, K., et al., Brief report: Asperger's syndrome and sibling birth order. Journal of Autism and Developmental Disorders, 2012.

[75] Keen, D., F. Reid, and D. Arnone, Autism, ethnicity and maternal immigration. British Journal of Psychiatry, 2010. 196: p. 274-81.

[76] Haglund, N. and K. Källén, Risk factors for autism and Asperger syndrome. Autism, 2011. 15(2): p. 163-83.

[77] Barnevik–Olsson, M., C. Gillberg, and E. Fernell, Prevalence of autism in children born to Somali parents living in Sweden: a brief report. Developmental Medicine and Child Neurology, 2008. 50(8): p. 598-601.

[78] Schieve, L., et al., Association between parental nativity and autism spectrum disorder among US-born non-Hispanic white and Hispanic children, 2007 National Survey of Children's Health. Disability and Health Journal, 2012. 5(1): p. 18-25.

[79] Fernell, E., et al., Serum levels of 25-hydroxyvitamin D in mothers of Swedish and of Somali origin who have children with and without autism. Acta Pædiatrica, 2010. 99(5): p. 743-7.

[80] Cannell, J., Autism and vitamin D. Medical Hypotheses, 2008. 70: p. 750-9.

[81] Zhou, M. and Y. Sao Xiong, The multifaceted American experiences of the children of Asian immigrants: lessons for segmented assimilation. Ethnic and Racial Studies, 2005. 28(6): p. 1119-52.

[82] Grulich, A., M. McCredie, and M. Coates, Cancer incidence in Asian migrants to New South Wales, Australia. British Journal of Cancer, 1995. 71(2): p. 400-8.

[83] Ip, D., C.-T. Wu, and C. Inglis, Settlement experiences of Taiwanese immigrants in Australia. Asian Studies Review, 1998. 22(1): p. 79-97.

[84] Pedersen, A., et al., Prevalence of autism spectrum disorders in Hispanic and non-Hispanic white children. Pediatrics, 2012.

[85] O'Leary, C., et al., Intellectual disability: population-based estimates of the proportion attributable to heavy prenatal alcohol exposure. Developmental Medicine and Child Neurology, 2012.

[86] O'Leary, C., Fetal alcohol syndrome: diagnosis, epidemiology and developmental outcomes. Journal of Paediatrics and Child Health, 2004. 40(1-2): p. 2-7.

[87] Wilson, K. and L. Watson, Autism spectrum disorder in Australian Indigenous families: issues of diagnosis, support and funding. Aboriginal and Islander Health Worker Journal, 2011. 35(5): p. 17-8.

[88] World Health Organisation. Mental health. 2012 [2012 September 3]; Available from: http://www.who.int/topics/mental_health/en/.

[89] Daniels, J., et al., Parental psychiatric disorders associated with autism spectrum disorders in the offspring. Pediatrics, 2008. 121(5): p. 1357-62.

[90] Mouridsen, S., et al., Psychiatric disorders in the parents of individuals with infantile autism: a case-control study. Psychopathology, 2007. 40(3): p. 166-71.

[91] Sullivan, P., et al., Family history of schizophrenia and bipolar disorder as risk factors for autism. Archives of General Psychiatry, 2012: p. 1-5.

[92] Zhang, X., et al., Prenatal and perinatal risk factors for autism in China. Journal of Autism and Developmental Disorders, 2010. 40(11): p. 1311-21.

[93] Wilkerson, D., et al., Perinatal complications as predictors of infantile autism. International Journal of Neuroscience, 2002. 112(9): p. 1085-98.

[94] Piven, J., et al., Psychiatric disorders in the parents of autistic individuals. Journal of the American Academy of Child and Adolescent Psychiatry, 1991. 30(3): p. 471-8.

[95] Morgan, V., et al., Intellectual disability and other neuropsychiatric outcomes in high-risk children of mothers with schizophrenia, bipolar disorder and unipolar major depression. British Journal of Psychiatry, 2012.

[96] Gokcen, S., et al., Theory of mind and verbal working memory deficits in parents of autistic children. Psychiatry Research, 2009. 166(1): p. 46-53.

[97] Hurley, R., et al., The broad autism phenotype questionnaire. Journal of Autism and Developmental Disorders, 2007. 37(9): p. 1679-90.

[98] Wong, D., et al., Profiles of executive function in parents and siblings of individuals with autism spectrum disorders. Genes, Brain and Behavior, 2006. 5(8): p. 561-76.

[99] Hughes, C., M. Leboyer, and M. Bouvard, Executive function in parents of children with autism. Psychological Medicine, 1997. 27(1): p. 209-20.

[100] Bishop, D., et al., Using self-report to identify the broad phenotype in parents of children with autistic spectrum disorders: a study using the Autism Spectrum Quotient. Journal of Child Psychology and Psychiatry, 2004. 45(8): p. 1431-6.

[101] Baron-Cohen, S., et al., The Autism Spectrum Quotient (AQ): evidence from Asperger syndrome/high-functioning autism, males and females, scientists and mathematicians. Journal of Autism and Developmental Disorders, 2001. 31(1): p. 5-17.

[102] Wheelwright, S., et al., Defining the broader, medium and narrow autism phenotype among parents using the Autism Spectrum Quotient (AQ). Molecular Autism, 2010. 1(1): p. 10.

[103] Bernier, R., et al., Evidence for broader autism phenotype characteristics in parents from multiple incidence autism families. Autism Research, 2011.

[104] Marques-Vidal, P., et al., Secular trends in height and weight among children and adolescents of the Seychelles, 1956-2006. BioMed Central Public Health, 2008. 8(1): p. 166.

[105] Kalkbrenner, A., et al., Maternal smoking during pregnancy and the prevalence of autism spectrum disorders, using data from the autism and developmental disabilities monitoring network. Environmental Health Perspectives, 2012. 120(7): p. 1042-8.

[106] Lee, B., et al., Brief report: maternal smoking during pregnancy and autism spectrum disorders. Journal of Autism and Developmental Disorders, 2011: p. 1-6.

[107] Braun, J., et al., The effect of maternal smoking during pregnancy on intellectual disabilities among 8 year old children. Paediatric and Perinatal Epidemiology, 2009. 23(5): p. 482-91.

[108] Spohr, H., J. Willms, and H. Steinhausen, Fetal alcohol spectrum disorders in young adulthood. Journal of Pediatrics, 2007. 150(2): p. 175-9.

[109] Spohr, H. and H. Steinhausen, Fetal alcohol spectrum disorders and their persisting sequelae in adult life. Deutsches Arzteblatt, 2008. 105(41): p. 693-8.

[110] Malbin, D., Fetal alcohol spectrum disorder (FASD) and the role of family court judges in improving outcomes for children and families. Juvenile and Family Court Journal, 2004. 55(2): p. 53-63.

[111] Hagberg, B. and M. Kyllerman, Epidemiology of mental retardation-a Swedish survey. Brain and Development, 1983. 5(5): p. 441-9.

[112] Yeargin-Allsopp, M., et al., Reported biomedical causes and associated medical conditions for mental retardation among 10 year old children, metropolitan Atlanta, 1985 to 1987. Developmental Medicine and Child Neurology, 1997. 39: p. 142-9.

[113] Quattlebaum, J. and M. O'Connor, Higher functioning children with prenatal alcohol exposure: Is there a specific neurocognitive profile? Child Neuropsychology, 2012: p. 1-18.

[114] Eyal, R. and M. O'Connor, Psychiatry trainees' training and experience in fetal alcohol spectrum disorders. Academic Psychiatry, 2011. 35: p. 238-40.

[115] Cnattingius, S., The epidemiology of smoking during pregnancy: smoking prevalence, maternal characteristics, and pregnancy outcomes. Nicotine and Tobacco Research, 2004. 6(Suppl 2): p. S125-S140.

[116] Naeye, R., Effects of maternal cigarette smoking on the fetus and placenta. British Journal of Obstetrics and Gynaecology, 1978. 85(10): p. 732-7.

[117] Wakschlag, L., et al., Maternal smoking during pregnancy and severe antisocial behavior in offspring: a review. American Journal of Public Health, 2002. 92(6): p. 966-72.

[118] Leonard, H., et al., Relation between intrauterine growth and subsequent intellectual disability in a ten-year population cohort of children in Western Australia. American Journal of Epidemiology, 2008. 167(1): p. 103-11.

[119] Ornoy, A. and Z. Ergaz, Alcohol abuse in pregnant women: effects on the fetus and newborn, mode of action and maternal treatment. International Journal of Environmental Research and Public Health, 2010. 7(2): p. 364-79.

[120] Lyall, K., et al., Maternal early life factors associated with hormone levels and the risk of having a child with an autism spectrum disorder in the Nurses Health Study II. Journal of Autism and Developmental Disorders, 2011. 41(5): p. 618-27.

[121] McLaren, L., Socioeconomic status and obesity. Epidemiologic Reviews, 2007. 29(1): p. 29-48.

[122] Mokdad, A., et al., The spread of the obesity epidemic in the United States, 1991-1998. Journal of the American Medical Association, 1999. 282(16): p. 1519-22.

[123] Comi, A., et al., Familial clustering of autoimmune disorders and evaluation of medical risk factors in autism. Journal of Child Neurology, 1999. 14(6): p. 388-94.

[124] Croen, L., et al., Maternal autoimmune diseases, asthma and allergies, and childhood autism spectrum disorders: a case-control study. Archives of Pediatrics and Adolescent Medicine, 2005. 159(2): p. 151-7.

[125] Atladóttir, H., et al., Association of family history of autoimmune diseases and autism spectrum disorders. Pediatrics, 2009. 124(2): p. 687-94.

[126] Mann, J., et al., Children born to diabetic mothers may be more likely to have intellectual disability. Maternal and Child Health Journal, 2012: p. 1-5.

[127] Leonard, H., et al., Maternal health in pregnancy and intellectual disability in the offspring: a population-based study. Annals of Epidemiology, 2006. 16(6): p. 448-54.

[128] Braunschweig, D., et al., Autism: maternally derived antibodies specific for fetal brain proteins. Neurotoxicology, 2008. 29(2): p. 226-31.

[129] Ashwood, P., S. Wills, and J. Van de Water, The immune response in autism: a new frontier for autism research. Journal of Leukocyte Biology, 2006. 80(1): p. 1-15.

[130] Goines, P., et al., Increased midgestational IFN-g, IL-4 and IL-5 in women bearing a child with autism: a case-control study. Molecular Autism, 2011. 2(13): p. e1-e11.

[131] Derecki, N., E. Privman, and J. Kipnis, Rett syndrome and other autism spectrum disorders-brain diseases of immune malfunction? Molecular Psychiatry, 2010. 15(4): p. 355-63.

[132] McDonough, J., Stedman's Concise Medical Dictionary, 1994: Williams & Wilkins.

[133] Rudra, C. and M. Williams, Monthly variation in preeclampsia prevalence: Washington State, 1987-2001. Journal of Maternal-Fetal and Neonatal Medicine, 2005. 18(5): p. 319-24.

[134] Mann, J., et al., Pre-eclampsia, birth weight, and autism spectrum disorders. Journal of Autism and Developmental Disorders, 2010. 40(5): p. 548-54.

[135] Griffith, M., J. Mann, and S. McDermott, The risk of intellectual disability in children born to mothers with preeclampsia or eclampsia with partial mediation by low birth weight. Hypertension in Pregnancy, 2011. 30(1): p. 108-15.

[136] Atladóttir, H., et al., Maternal infection requiring hospitalization during pregnancy and autism spectrum disorders. Journal of Autism and Developmental Disorders, 2010. 40(12): p. 1423-30.

[137] Mann, J., et al., Trichomoniasis in pregnancy and mental retardation in children. Annals of Epidemiology, 2009. 19(12): p. 891-99

[138] McDermott, S., et al., Urinary tract infections during pregnancy and mental retardation and developmental delay. Obstetrics and Gynecology, 2000. 96(1): p. 113-9.

[139] Croen, L., et al., Antidepressant use during pregnancy and childhood autism spectrum disorders. Archives of General Psychiatry, 2011. 68(11): p. 11104-12.

[140] Rasalam, A., et al., Characteristics of fetal anticonvulsant syndrome associated autistic disorder. Developmental Medicine and Child Neurology, 2005. 47(8): p. 551-5.

[141] Maimburg, R. and M. Væth, Perinatal risk factors and infantile autism. Acta Psychiatrica Scandinavica, 2006. 114(4): p. 257-64.

Chapter 2

Co-Occurrence of Developmental Disorders: Children Who Share Symptoms of Autism, Dyslexia and Attention Deficit Hyperactivity Disorder

Ginny Russell and Zsuzsa Pavelka

Additional information is available at the end of the chapter

1. Introduction

Children with autism spectrum disorders (ASD) have a higher risk of suffering from several other conditions. In this chapter I review the extent to which autistic individuals can also experience a range of other difficulties, but my focus will be on the common neurodevelopmental disorders. The most common of these include dyslexia, attention deficit hyperactivity disorder (ADHD), dyspraxia, specific language impairment, and dyscalculia. There is considerable symptom overlap in particular between ADHD and dyslexia, and like autism both are described as developmental disorders by psychiatric classification systems (American Psychiatric Association, 2000; World Health Organization., 1992). Overlapping conditions are termed 'co-morbidity' by medical practitioners. Co-morbidity may reflect the greater difficulties experienced by children with a combination of deficits. Sometimes it is apparent that many children with a developmental disorder could be classified in several ways. Here I will firstly examine the research evidence that examines how often symptoms of dyslexia and ADHD occur in the population of autistic children, and second, review the various theories that have tried to explain why such co-occurring difficulties are so common.

'Comorbidity', a term used in medical literature to mean a dual diagnosis, or multiple diagnoses, can reflect an inability to supply a single diagnosis that accounts for all symptoms. Children with ASD have been shown to have higher rates of epilepsy, with 30% of cases having epilepsy comorbid (Danielsson, Gillberg, Billstedt, Gillberg, & Olsson, 2005). Other conditions that are commonly co-morbid with ASD include hearing impairment (Kielinen, Rantala, Timonen, Linna, & Moilanen, 2004) mental health and behavioural problems (Bradley, Summers, Wood, & Bryson, 2004), including anxiety, and depression (Evans, Canavera,

Kleinpeter, Maccubbin, & Taga, 2005). It has also been shown that parents of autistic children are twice as likely themselves to have suffered from psychiatric illness than parents of non-autistic children (Daniels et al., 2008).

Most of these problems are distinct from those examined in this chapter: the common developmental disorders of childhood which are also found to co-occur with autism, particularly ADHD and dyslexia.

Before reviewing the evidence that suggests many children share difficulties symptomatic of these conditions, and the theories of why this may be, I will briefly describe how dyslexia and ADHD manifest themselves.

2. Dyslexia

Dyslexia is conceptualized by both educational bodies and the psychiatric classification systems as a learning difficulty that primarily affects the skills involved in accurate and fluent word reading and spelling. Characteristic features of dyslexia are difficulties in phonological awareness, verbal memory and verbal processing speed. Dyslexia is developmental delay in literacy and generally slow and inaccurate reading and spelling. The definition of dyslexia has changed over time, and such changes have often been based on the research identifying a range of associated difficulties that occur with dyslexia. Estimates of the prevalence of dyslexia have been complicated because dyslexia cut-offs are contested (Coltheart & Jackson, 1998) and dyslexia manifests itself differently in various languages according to levels of phonic regularity (Miles, 2004). Research over the last 40 years has focused on phonological skills. These are the reading and de-coding skills used when breaking down language into its component sounds and reassembling the parts in order to read or to spell a word.

Like autism, dyslexic difficulties are considered to exist in a continuum throughout the general population (Fawcett, 2012). There is much interest in the association of cognitive ability with changing symptom profiles and diagnosis. The definition of dyslexia is in flux, and has been recently redefined by many national bodies, for example in the UK, the British Psychological Society, focusing on literacy learning at the 'word level' without attainment discrepancy:

Dyslexia is evident when accurate and fluent word reading and/or spelling develops very incompletely or with great

difficulty (British Psychological Society, 1999)

This definition implies that the problem is severe and persistent despite appropriate learning opportunities. This UK definition differs from the ICD-10 diagnosis of developmental dyslexia or 'Specific Reading Disorder', which requires a discrepancy between actual reading ability and the reading ability predicted by a child's IQ. So an intellectual disability, (generally considered IQ below 70) can co-occur with the British Psychological Society definition of dyslexia. This new definition includes the so called 'garden variety' dyslexic children who have difficulties with reading and spelling as well as other generalized intellectual disabilities. The implications of including this group as dyslexic mean that more children with an intellectual disability would also be classified as 'dyslexic'. As ASD includes a large group with intellectual disability the extension is likely to increase the number of children who may be classified as having both conditions. This is important as the clinical and education label may determine the interventions a particular child receives.

In addition to these characteristics, dyslexic children may experience visual and auditory processing difficulties, similar to hyper or hypo sensitivity often associated with ASD. Like the 'islets of ability' seen in many children with ASD, some dyslexic children may also have strengths in particular areas, such as design, logic, and creative skills.

3. ADHD

ADHD is known as 'Hyperkinetic Disorder' in ICD-10; there are three subtypes of ADHD according the DSM. In the first, a child will primarily have problems with attention which may manifest as an inability to remain 'on task' for long periods, lack of response to instruction or distractibility. In the second sub-type, symptoms of hyperactivity and impulsivity dominate, which is characterized by wriggling, squirming, being unable to sit still, interrupting and finding it difficult to wait. Children may also be climbing in inappropriate situations and always on the move when free to do so. The third sub-type is simply the co-existence of both attention problems and hyperactivity, with each behavior occurring infrequently alone and symptoms starting before seven years of age.

According to ICD-10, eventually, assessment instruments should develop to the point where it is possible to take a quantitative cut-off score to assess ADHD. Like dyslexia and autism, the symptoms are behavioural in nature, and are part of a continuously distributed pattern that extends into the population at large.

The persistence of ADHD symptoms is not so marked as for autism. Around 70 to 50 percent of those individuals diagnosed in childhood do not continue to have symptoms into adulthood (Elia, Ambrosini, & Rapoport, 1999). There is evidence suggesting to some extent symptoms of ADHD are expressed in reaction to home (Mulligan et al. 2011) and other environmental contexts. Individuals with ADHD also tend to develop coping mechanisms to compensate for some or all of their impairments. ADHD is diagnosed more often in boys with the reported ratio varying from 2:1 to 4:1 (Dulcan, 1997; Kessler et al., 2005) though some studies suggest this may be partially due to referral bias where teachers are more likely to refer boys than girls (Sciutto, Nolfi, & Bluhm, 2004). Treatments for ADHD involve a combination of medication, usually methyphenidates which are well established in improving symptoms of inattention, and behavioral intervention in education and at home. The issue of girls being overlooked on identification is a common thread for research in dyslexia, ADHD and autism. Our own results suggest there is some evidence to back up the claim that boys with ASD symptoms are given the diagnosis more frequently than girls with equivalent ASD symptoms (Russell, Steer, & Golding, 2011). This may be because the disorders tend to be conceptualized as 'male' leading to referral bias.

Because ASD, Dyslexia and ADHD are all behaviorally defined, so 'symptoms' are behaviours. All three conditions are conceived as particular behaviours along a spectrum, where traits have a continuous distribution and extend into the general (non-disordered) population. An arbitrary cut off point determines who is considered to be within the various categories and who is not. The clinician giving a diagnosis will be responsible for judging where this cut off may come, guided by diagnostic criteria and standards within disciplines as well as perceived implications: the benfits versus any possible risks of assigning a diagnosis. This is perhaps best established for autism: Constantino and Todd (2003) measured autistic traits in a large community sample, and found no jump in the threshold of autistic behaviours between 'normal' individuals and those with an autism spectrum diagnosis, rather they found a continuous distribution. These findings concurred with those in a Scandinavian study (Posserud, Lundervold, & Gillberg, 2006). One of our own studies has likewise shown that autistic traits do extend into the 'subclinical' population (Figure 1). As with dyslexia and ADHD, there is not a sharp line separating severity in those with a diagnosis from less severe traits in those without (London, 2007). In both dyslexia, ADHD and the autism spectrum, some children have more severe difficulties than others, and the symptoms extend into the population of children (and adults) as a whole. For dyslexia, there are many people who may have mild dyslexic difficulties but perhaps might not qualify as 'dyslexic'. For autism spectrum disorders, many people without an autism diagnosis do have autistic-type behaviours but the severity and frequency of those behavioural symptoms is less severe than in those deemed to qualify for a diagnosis.

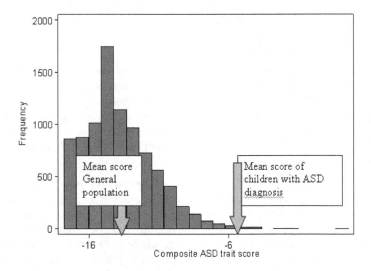

Figure 1. The distribution of an ASD composite trait in the general population from Russell et al.(2012)

The imposition of a cut off between normality and abnormality is therefore 'an arbitrary but convenient way of converting a dimension into a category' as Goodman and Scott (1997, p. 23) point out.

4. Evidence of symptom overlap – ASD and ADHD

Various studies have looked for ADHD or ADHD symptoms in samples of children with autism or ASD. Rates of ADHD have ranged from 28% to 78% of these samples (Ronald, Edelson, Asherson, & Saudino, 2010). Studies that look at ADHD symptoms have reported even higher numbers: for example, Sturm, Fernell, & Gillberg, (2004) looked at a sample of around 100 high functioning children with ASD and found 95% had attention problems, 75% had motor difficulties, 86% had problems with regulation of activity level, and 50% had impulsiveness. About three-quarters had symptoms compatible with mild or severe ADHD, or had deficits in attention, motor control, and perception, indicating a considerable overlap between these disorders and high-functioning ASD in children.

In an large analysis of nine hundred forty-six twins, Reierson and colleagues (2008) assigned DSM-IV ADHD diagnoses, and measured autistic traits using the Social Responsiveness Scale. The study showed that there are clinically significant elevations of autistic traits in children meeting diagnostic criteria for ADHD. These findings confirm results in earlier studies (Clark, Feehan, Tinline, & Vostanis, 1999). Santosh and Mijoovic (2004) which found children with ADHD had elevated levels of impairment in all three autistic symptom domains, namely social deficits, communication and stereotyped behaviors. Clark *et al* found 65-80% of parents of children with ADHD reported difficulties in social interaction (particularly in empathy and peer relationships) and in communication (particularly in imagination, and maintaining conversation). So the presence of autistic traits in children with ADHD appears common (Ronald et al., 2010).

In an analysis conducted with Lauren Rodgers at the Peninsula Medical School in the UK using data from the Millennium Cohort Study, a cohort of around 19,000 children who were all born between 2000 and 2002, we noted 44 children had a dual diagnosis of both ASD and ADHD (proportion of total population 0.3%) by age seven. The prevalence of children with identified ADHD in the ASD sample was 17%. Conversely, the prevalence of children with ASD in the ADHD sample was higher at 27%. Both figures indicate substantial overlap between these conditions.

Various European research groups have examined co-morbid disorders in adults with diagnosed ASD. An international team lead by Hofvander studied a group of 122 adults with normal IQ from specialist clinics in three European cities: Gothenburg, Paris and Malmö (Hofvander et al., 2009). Here the overwhelming majority had symptoms of ASD. Nonverbal communication problems were also very common, described in 89% of all their subjects. In this study over half the participants, (52%) were diagnosed with co-morbid ADHD. Interestingly, participants diagnosed with pervasive developmental disorder. 'Not Otherwise Specified' (PDD-NOS) diagnosis had significantly more symptoms of inattention and hyperactivity/impulsivity compared to subjects diagnosed with Asperger's syndrome. However, the prevalence of the categorical diagnosis of ADHD did not differ significantly between the groups, nor were gender differences apparent. Although the study presents clear evidence of many cases where patients display symptoms of both ADHD and ASD, the clinical setting may have led to selection bias as patients with complex needs may be more likely to seek help.

Because behaviours associated with both conditions lie on a spectrum extending into the normal range, some studies have found a range of frequency and severity of symptoms. In Mulligan et al.'s (2009) study, for example, 75 of children with ADHD had severe autism traits, and over half showed sub-clinical autism symptoms. Kadesjö and colleagues (Kadesjö, Gillberg, & Hagberg, 1999), looked at comorbidity of ADHD in Swedish school-age children and found only 1% of children meeting the threshold for ADHD had comorbid Aspergers Syndrome (AS). The estimates of co-morbidity of ADHD symptoms with ASD symptoms vary widely because of differing methods of case ascertainment. An additional problem is that the estimate of the prevalence of ASD itself has increased so much in western countries, making ASD itself a 'moving target' (Figure 2).

Patricia Howlin (2000) reviewed the estimated rates of co-existing psychiatric disorders in subjects with high functioning ASD and found these estimates varied from 9% to 89% - very substantial differences. However it is possible to generalise; thirty years of research have confirmed that attention deficits and hyperactivity are relatively common in children and adults with ASD even if the exact extent of overlap is dependent on methodology and ascertainment (Hofvander et al., 2009, Sturm, Fernell, & Gillberg, 2004).

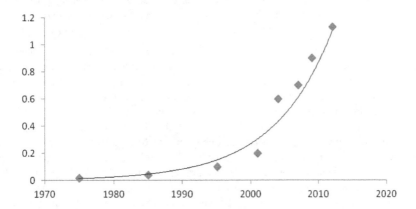

Figure 2. The rising prevalence of autism spectrum disorders over 50 years. (Data from 'Autism Speaks' and CDC, USA)

Recent trends have made categorical diagnosis an integral part of everyday clinical and research practice (Sonuga-Barke & Halperin, 2010). Christopher Gillberg (2010) points out that clinicians have become focused on dichotomous categories of disorder and that clinics have become increasingly specialized and overlook difficulties not within their immediate jurisdiction. Gillberg has argued that co-existence of disorders is the rule rather than the exception in child psychiatry and developmental medicine. He has coined the acronym ESSENCE (referring to Early Symptomatic Syndromes Eliciting

Neurodevelopmental Clinical Examinations). This describes cases where a combination of symptoms including inattention, hyperactivity, social and reading difficulties are observed. Major problems in at least one ESSENCE domain before age 5 years often signal major problems in the same or overlapping domains years later.

To summarize, although ADHD and ASD are separate and recognizable, there is good evidence that these conditions co-occur, constituting an amalgam of problems.

5. Comorbidity between dyslexia and ASD

There is only a small literature on the overlap in symptomology between autism spectrum disorders with those of dyslexia. Officially, as for ADHD, ASD is an exclusionary criterion for diagnosis of dyslexia and vice versa, but ASD also shows overlap with dyslexia in both cognitive and behavioural features (Reiersen & Todd, 2008, Simonoff et al., 2008). A proportion of children share symptoms between dyslexia, ADHD *and* ASD.

The number of children that do share symptoms of ASD and dyslexia is likely to be small (Wright, Conlon, Wright, & Dyck, 2011). The frequency of reading disorder in combination with disorder of written expression (i.e. dyslexia) was around 14% in a sample of adults with Asperger's Syndrome (AS) so according to this result around one in seven individuals with AS will have co-occurring dyslexia (Hofvander et al., 2009). However the proportion of individuals with dyslexia who have co-occuring AS is likely to be low as Asperger's Syndrome is much a rarer condition than dyslexia.

A common problem for children with dyslexia is misinterpretation of spoken language, which can also manifest itself in comprehension. This produces further overlap with pragmatic language impairment (PLI) which itself is virtually indistinguishable from communication difficulties associated with high functioning autism. Pragmatic language difficulties may involve literal interpretation so 'run on the spot' would have a child looking for a big black spot to run on, for example. Children with PLI will often fail to interpret the core meaning or saliency of events. This causes a penchant for routine and 'sameness' (also seen in autism and Asperger's Syndrome) as PLI children struggle to generalize and take hold of the meaning of novel situations. Obvious and concrete instructions are clearly understood and carried out, whereas simple but non-literal expressions such as jokes, sarcasm and general social chatting are difficult and may be misinterpretated. PLI may therefore impact on the social abilities of the child who has difficulty interpreting jokes. Current thinking is that PLI is not a problem rooted in language skills but one of social communication and information processing. Griffiths (2007) identified difficulties of this type in dyslexic students, showed they were impaired in making inferences from a story and choosing the right punch-line for a joke. This of course can have implications for written language and examinations under stress, as well as for a range of social interactions.

It is not just that ASD is co-morbid with dyslexia and ADHD. Other studies have noted high comorbidity with other developmental disorders. Dyspraxia and dyscalculia and conditions with shared symptoms such as specific language impairment are frequently comorbid with autism. Also dyslexia and ADHD themselves co-occur Willcutt and colleagues (Willcutt, Doyle, Nigg, Faraone, & Pennington, 2005) showed that 40% of a sample of twins with either dyslexia or ADHD was co-morbid for the other disorder. Reading difficulties were measured with both rating scale and an objective task in a study by Cheung et al. (2012) and correlations were observed among ADHD, reading difficulties and IQ. Over half, (53%-72%) of the overlapping familial influences between ADHD and reading difficulties were not shared with IQ. In a school based study Kadesjö and colleagues found 40% of children with ADHD showed reading problems and 29% writing problems (2005).

Overall, the literature suggests, there is good evidence to suggest that some children do suffer from symptoms of both dyslexia and ASD, although this is not so well established, and does not occur so frequently as co-morbidity between ADHD and ASD.

6. Reasons for co-occurrence of ASD with other developmental disorders

Several theories have been put forward to explain the shared symptoms of the various developmental conditions – in other words why specific learning and language and social disorders are not specific. It is likely that all the explanations below play a part in co-occurrence; the causality of co-morbidity is most probably due to a complex web of interacting factors.

7. Genetic explanations

One of the most persuasive explanations is that a genetic predisposition may lead to abnormal neurological development, which in turn may manifest in various different aberrant behaviors and developmental delays. As autism, ADHD and dyslexia and other developmental conditions are all highly heritable, so they all have a large genetic component, the theory seems plausible. The same genetic anomaly may lead to several disorders or psychiatric conditions. In other words one genotype may lead to several (related) phenotypes. This is known as 'pleiotropy'. Researchers have suggested that co-occurrence of autism and ADHD (and other developmental disorders) may reflect such common genetic causes (Reierson et al, 2008). In this model, the origins of both sets of difficulties are due to common genetic anomalies that predispose children to delayed or atypical neurological development. Certainly, specific genetic anomalies have been associated with a range of psychopathologies in adulthood. However, the genetic picture is complex and exact pathways are not established. It is estimated there are more than a thousand gene variations which could disrupt brain development enough to result in social delays (Sanders et al., 2012).

Such a genetic predisposition is almost certainly complex and multi factorial. So far, over 100 candidate genes have been associated with ASD, most of which encode proteins involved in neural development, but exact mutations within the candidate genes have yet to be identified (Freitag, 2007). Furthermore, different individuals may have mutations in different sets of genes and most of the discovered gene variations are likely to have a low penetrance, thus not all carriers will develop the disorder. There may be interactions among mutations in several genes, e.g. between regulatory genes and coding regions, or between the environment and mutated genes, altering their expression. The effect of a mutation or deletion can depend on processes relating to gene expression and regulation as well as the subsequent effects on the expression of other genes.

The advent of genomics and the emphasis placed on this has led to much research to identify genetic predispositions to ASD. The field of psychiatry as a whole has been 'geneticised' according to some social theorists. This refers to the potential reclassification of psychiatric conditions in the light of findings from molecular biology. For example, a particular sub-category of DSM-IV schizophrenia has been linked to a substitution of a single base in the sequence of DNA of a particular gene localised to a precise place on a particular chromosome, leading to a substitution of one amino-acid for another in an enzyme involved in neurotransmission. Hedgecoe (2001) provides a discussion of the geneticisation of schizophrenia. The debate as to whether the old psychiatric systems of classification should be overhauled in the light of new genomic knowledge which illuminates genetic aetiologies is ongoing (Ericson & Doyle, 2003).

8. Gene-environment interactions

A second theory is that an environmental insult or a stressful event in the life of the fetus or in a young child's life, may trigger a genetic predisposition to be expressed. Thus this constitutes a gene- environmental interaction theory. An example might be the high testosterone levels in the womb that have been observed in some studies. Baron-Cohen's Cambridge group, for example, has carried out work that has suggested high levels of fetal testosterone may be linked to the development of autistic traits (Ingudomnukul, Baron-Cohen, Wheelwright, & Knickmeyer, 2007). According to the gene-environment explanation, the elevated testosterone might lead to the differential expression of genes controlling the neurological development of the child. Another example that has been quite widely publicized concerns Omega 3 fatty acids. These have been implicated by Richardson (2006), who has argued that attention-deficit/hyperactivity disorder, dyslexia, developmental coordination disorder (dyspraxia) and conditions on the autism spectrum may all share common origins triggered by problems with phospholipid (fatty acid) metabolism. However this is just one genetic / environmental explanation for co-occurrence that vies with several others, and the available evidence is subject to interpretation.

In the majority of cases, the gene-environment hypothesis seems highly plausible. It may be that autism and co-occurring developmental conditions may all be caused by a genetic predisposition which is triggered by an early environmental influence (Trottier, Srivastava, & Walker, 1999).

Many environmental factors have been implicated in ASD but the effect of each is poorly established. After the well publicized paper that linked autism to the MMR vaccination, research has repeatedly refuted a link between the MMR jab and ASD (Rutter, 2005). Deykin and MacMahon (1979) found increased risk due to exposure to, and clinical illness from, common viral illnesses in the first 18 months of life. In this study, mumps, chickenpox, fever of unknown origin, and ear infections were all significantly associated with ASD risk. Epidemiological studies have shown there is a higher rate of adverse prenatal and postnatal events in children with ASD than in the general population (Zwaigenbaum et al., 2002). Newschaffer and colleague's (2007) review named associated obstetric conditions that included low birth weight, gestation duration, and caesarean section. It is possible that such an underlying cause partially could explain both autism and the associated conditions (Kolevzon, Gross, & Reichenberg, 2007). There is evidence to suggest adverse prenatal and perinatal events are also associated with ADHD and cognitive development. Some studies have suggested that the risk of autism may be increased with advancing maternal age (Bolton et al., 1997). Paternal age too has frequently (but not always) associated with autism. There are more mutations in the gametes of older men, and this higher rate of mutation in the genetic material from the paternal side may explain the higher levels of neurodevelopmental disabilities in their offspring. An alternative explanation is that fathers who themselves have autistic traits are less likely to have children young. Using anticonvulsants during pregnancy also appears to increase the risk of ASD (Moore et al., 2000). These drugs are used to combat epilepsy which is commonly often comorbid with ASD. Parental occupational exposure to chemicals during the preconception period has also been higher in ASD families than controls in some studies (Felicetti, 1981).

Environmental risk factors have received widespread media coverage within the last few years, perhaps because of the strong degree of public concern (Russell & Kelly, 2011). In most health and disease categories, a secondary function of diagnosis is to group together people who have a common aetiology. However, the specific effects of genetic factors and environmental risk factors that might play a part in abnormal neural development are largely unresolved. Goodman and Scott (1997) stress that current understanding of aetiology for childhood developmental conditions will probably look ridiculously simplistic or misguided in years to come. Despite, or perhaps because of, the uncertainty, there is an underlying concern among people involved with children who are diagnosed with developmental conditions that environmental influences may be partially to blame for rising incidence. Novel prenatal and perinatal medical practices, changing diet, shifting family structures and childhood social activities have all been the subject of lay theories to explain rising prevalence not just of ASD, but developmental disorders in childhood more generally, including ADHD and dyslexia (Russell & Kelly, 2011).

9. The influence of childcare and the child's environment

A third possibility is that environmental factors alone may be enough to trigger not just autistic behaviors, but also other maladaptive behaviors such as inattention. Autistic behaviors were observed in a study of abandoned Romanian children, conducted by Michael Rutter and colleagues (1999). As well as cases with known genetic causes, in some cases, underlying social factors may predispose autistic symptoms. In this study, Rutter and colleagues noted a very high instance of autism (6%) in the Romanian baby cohort, which they put down to poor early care. These children exhibited typical symptoms of autism at four years old, but unlike cases of autism without maltreatment, symptoms by age 6 were much milder. This case is an illustration of how children who share severe autistic symptoms at young ages may have differing developmental trajectories. In this study, the symptoms of autism may have been triggered primarily by the early neglect, rather than by a genetic predisposition, for if a genetic predisposition was involved it would effect 6% or more of the babies, a very high proportion.

It is not just aetiological environmental factors that seem to lead to increased risks of displaying autistic behaviours. Aetiological causes can be distinguished from proximate determinates which occur at the same time as symptoms, for example, social situations or fluorescent lights may exacerbate the expression of ASD symptoms. There are also those influences in the environment that are sometimes referred to in psychiatry as maintenance factors, including stigmatisation and labelling. Although their influence in perpetuating ASD and other developmental disorders is unclear, an influence in maintaining symptomatic behaviours of autism and co-morbid conditions can not be discounted. Biological causes and behavioural outcomes are mediated by experiential and environmental factors.

10. Cognitive causes and developmental consequences

The competing psychological theories that have been put forward concerning the psychological mechanisms of ASD include weak central coherence theory, deficits in executive function and the extreme male brain theory, all were reviewed by Happé in 1994.

The extreme male brain theory as developed by Baron-Cohen (2002) suggests that autistic individuals can systematize—that is, they can develop internal rules of operation—but are less effective at empathizing and handling events that are unexpected or social. The theory was developed from the earlier 'theory of mind' (Baron-Cohen, Leslie, & Frith, 1985). This suggested that autistic people lack the ability to understand other peoples' mental states, put themselves in another person's place or imagine what they might be thinking or experiencing. This lack of mentalising is discussed by Frith and Happé in their discussion of dyslexia, autism and downstream effects of specific impairments (1998). The 'theory of mind' lines up with the 'mirror neuron theory of autism' (Iacoboni & Dapretto, 2006) which was based on the discovery that the macaque monkey brain contained 'mirror neurons' that fired not only when the animal is in action, but also when it observes others carrying out the same actions.

An alternative psychological theory for autism is provided by Frith whose 'weak central coherence' theory (Frith, 2003; Happé & Frith, 2006) describes the ability to place information in a context in order to give it meaning. Most people pull together numerous stimuli to form a coherent picture of the world, allowing them to see the 'bigger picture'. In central coherence theory, the failure to appreciate the whole accounts for the piecemeal way in which people with ASD acquire knowledge. People with ASD may also show relative strengths in some areas, known as 'islets of ability'; and this accounts for savant skills. Related to central coherence is the theory that autistic behaviours are due to interference in executive function (Hill, 2004). Executive functions coordinate the flow of information processing in the brain and are the mechanisms of transferring attention from one thing to another flexibly and easily. They allow people to plan strategically, solve problems and set objectives. Their absence means autistic people show an inability to plan and attain overarching goals. This manifests as easily distractible behaviour and reliance on routines. Such psychological theories of ASD are useful models but have also been subject to criticism. Bailey and Parr (2003) describe such theories of psychological mechanisms as 'narrow cognitive conceptualisations' (p. 27), because they cannot accommodate the presence of sub-clinical autistic traits in the general population.

These theories seem very distinct from some psychological theories that explain dyslexic type and attention and hyperactive difficulties. The exception to this is that, deficits in executive function have been suggested as causal for ADHD, as they affect both cognitive and motivational systems (Willcutt et al., 2005). Frith and Happé (1998) focusing on dyslexia and autism, argue that psychological mechanisms could act as 'gateways' to impairment in other domains. These downstream developmental effects have not yet been fully considered, they suggest. Although they focus on autism and dyslexia, ADHD and other developmental disorders could easily be included in their model. As they point out, both dyslexia and autism have genetic origins, an anatomical basis and extremely variable behavioral manifestations. Their idea is that in addition to the genetic and anatomical origins, an additional developmental pathway may contribute to later difficulties. They argue that specific impairments seen in dyslexia or autism (such as dyslexic phonological or autistic mentalising difficulties) may have a 'gatekeeping' function and subsequently lead to difficulties in other areas. Thus impairments in domain-specific functions may have wide ranging developmental effects.

The idea put simply is that during development, one behavior exacerbates problems in other domains. It is perhaps easier to understand given a few concrete examples. Frith and Happé suggest that the core autistic difficulty of social engagement may lead to missed opportunities for learning, including learning vocabulary. This may effect language acquisition and in turn the development of language based skills evident in dyslexia. An easier pathway to understand might be via gatekeeping function of inattention. If a child is inattentive (a core symptom of ADHD) then the likelihood is they may struggle to focus on learning to read. Hence difficulties symptomatic of dyslexia may be expected. Conversely perhaps reading difficulties are primary, in which case inattention might come from frustration and inability to deal with task demands. This direction of causality seems likely in the sub-group of ADHD children whose problems only appear at school, and who are more likely than other groups to show reading problems according to Taylor (2011). Furthermore, an inattentive child may find it difficult to socialize normally, and may have difficulties following instruction. This may lead to the impairment in social skills symptomatic of autism.

In a similar way, it is possible to theorize that each domain of behavioural impairment in the triad for autism might lead to another. In a review of evidence for single genetic or cognitive causes for autism, Happé, Ronald, and Plomin (2006) note that twin studies suggest combinations of largely non-overlapping genes act on each area of impairment. Their own study found only modest correlations between the three domains of behavioural traits in the triad (namely deficits in social skills and communication and stereotyped behaviour or restricted interests). In the general population, correlations ranged from 0.1- 0.4 for the relationship of each domain to the other. This evidence shows that the three types of autistic traits may be clustered or linked or co-inherited, but with a weak association. These low correlations could be attributed to developmental pathways factors as well as genetic links. Such residual downstream developmental effects are easy to conceptualise. If a young boy is very asocial for example, then his communication skills will not be practised with peers, so he is unlikely to develop as quickly in measures of communication as a more sociable child. The weak correlation between repetitive behaviours is harder to explain. Speculation is possible: repetitive behaviours have been shown to have both self-stimulatory as well as calming functions (Turner, 1999). Repetitive behaviours can therefore be interpreted as responses to unwanted stimuli, e.g. social stimuli with which autistic people have difficulty. Williams (1994) has given a first person account of use of repetitive behaviours to ameliorate the stress of social situations. Conversely, the need for stimulatory repetitive behaviours, concentrating on drawing lines or circles for example, may interfere with social opportunities. Weak associations do not confirm or deny genetic co-inheritance. Developmental pathways where one type of behaviour leads to another may also provide a partial explanation.

In a different but related developmental scenario, Cheslack-Postava and Jordan –Young (2012) suggest that a child's upbringing is highly gendered, and proposed a gendered embodiment model for autism. They cite numerous studies illustrating that the nature of parenting in particular depends on the gender of the child. This they use to describe a gendered theory of development of autism, although the model could also explain the large predominance of boys with other developmental disorders. Cooper (2001) suggests boys are socialized to encourage competition and activity thus a conflict between passivity required at western schools and masculine identity is generated. Some behaviours associated with ADHD when used excessively in school environments, climbing trees for example, are encouraged more often in boys than girls. Cheslack-Postava and Jordan –Young suggest such gendered social processes interact with biology to promote certain 'disordered' behaviours. This they call the 'pervasive developmental environment'.

As well as downstream developmental models, some theorists have suggested one cognitive deficit may underlie several symptomatic behaviours. Although the cognitive/psychological theories of dyslexia and autism seem quite distinct, some research does suggest children with both ADHD and dyslexic difficulties show a distinctive deficit in rapid naming speed, so it may that processing speed underlies the link (Bental & Tirosh, 2007).

A second example is provided by executive function which is impaired in both autism and ADHD (Willcutt et al, 2005). According to some models, an underlying impairment in executive function prevents children from coordinating information processing in the brain, and

Co-Occurrence of Developmental Disorders: Children Who Share Symptoms of Autism, Dyslexia and Attention Deficit Hyperactivity Disorder

53

prevents the transfer attention from one thing to another. It is easy to understand how this absence may translate into symptoms of either autism, due to inability to plan with strategic overarching vision, and hence reliance on routines, or as inattention and distractibility symptomatic of ADHD. Executive functions are neuropsychological processes needed to sustain problem-solving toward a goal. Executive functions allow a resolution of conflict when two responses are simultaneously called for by stimuli. In the laboratory, the Stroop task is an example. The conflicting combination of a word like *red* written in green ink creates conflict when the task is to say the color of the ink (green), due to the overlearned reading response that automatically elicits the response based on the meaning of the word (red). Executive function allows for the inhibition of the overlearned response and the execution of a response that is more appropriate given the context. Research has confirmed the involvement of deficits in executive functions that are essential for effective self-regulation in people with ADHD. The mental processes most often listed as being part of the notion of executive function are quite diverse so there is no standardized definition. They include: inhibition, resistance to distraction, self-awareness, working memory, emotional self-control, and even self-motivation. Bramham and colleagues (2009) found that both adults with ASD and ADHD had impaired executive function, although they did have distinctive profiles. Nyden and colleagues found that children with Asperger's Syndrome and dyslexia did not differ in tests of executive function: they could not establish any test of executive function that captured the differences in these disorders (1999).

Russell Barkley (2012) conceptualizes executive control as the methods of self-regulation. He writes entertainingly on how a person might use executive functions to resist the temptation to buy a tempting pastry from a shop:

...avert your eyes from the counter, walk to a different section of the shop away from the tempting goodies, engage yourself in mental conversation about why you need to not buy those products, and even visualize an image of the new slenderer version of yourself you expect to achieve in the near future. All of these are self-directed actions you are using to try and alter the likelihood of giving into temptation and therefore increase your chances of meeting your goal of weight loss this month. This situation calls upon a number of distinct yet interacting mental abilities to successfully negotiate the situation. You have to be aware that a dilemma has arisen when you walked into the shop (self-awareness), you have to restrain your urge to order the pastry to go with the coffee you have ordered (inhibition), you redirected your attention away from the tempting objects (executive attention or attentional management), you spoke to yourself using your mind's voice (verbal self-instruction or working memory), and you visualized an image of your goal and what you would look like when you successfully attain it (nonverbal working memory, or visual imagery). You may also have found yourself thinking about various other ways you could have coped effectively with these temptations (problem-solving), and may have even used words of encouragement toward yourself to enhance the like-

lihood that you would follow your plan (self-motivation).

Barkley explains that these and other mental activities are usually included in the under-standing of human self-regulation, and it is difficulties in these areas (which are processes in executive function) that may lead to ADHD. Children with ADHD are distractible and self-regulation, the ability to override incoming stimuli, to see the bigger picture and lack the ability to see the consequences of their future actions. Children with ASD have difficulties transferring attention from one thing to another because they also lack overview (and impli-cations of their actions in the future).

Gooch, Snowling and Hulme (2011) note that deficits in time perception (the ability to judge the length of time intervals) have been found in children with both dyslexia and ADHD. These researchers found children with comorbid dyslexia and attention problems performed poorly on measures of executive function as well as on phonological tasks. However, their results were interpreted as the effect of independent underlying cognitive causes. Although deficits in duration discrimination were associated with both dyslexia and attention prob-lems, they concluded the results supported the claim that the two disorders are products of different cognitive defects originating from shared genes with pleiotropic effects.

Developmental models explain comorbidity of developmental disorders by shared cognitive deficits, either as 'gateways' as in Frith and Happés (1998) model, where one difficulty leads to another later in life, or as underlying shared deficits, for example impaired executive function causing both autism and ADHD. The alternative model suggests that cognitive dif-ficulties associated with each disorder are distinct, but multiple cognitive deficits arise from similar genetic/environmental origins. All these theories have some empirical support.

11. Diagnostic substitution and the influence of society and culture

When symptoms of two or more conditions are shared, whatever the psychological mecha-nisms (whether or not there are shared underlying cognitive deficits, and /or genetic and neurological differences) then the area of functioning that is highlighted as a problem may depend on which tests are administered. In our recent research we followed a six year old child who was assessed by three educational psychologists and one multidisciplinary team, each blind to the findings of the others. One concluded that the child had dyspraxia, two that the child had dyslexic difficulties, and a third that borderline AS was likely. We inter-preted these differences in the use of diagnostic labels as dependent on settings that varied during assessments, and assessment methods that exposed different types of behaviour (Russell, Norwich, & Gwernan-Jones, 2012). This work suggests that which diagnosis is as-signed depends to some extent on social and cultural factors as well as actual symptoms. If a child has symptoms of several disorders, then one context or test may draw out symptoms associated with one disorder, whereas another setting may expose symptoms of another.

Thus for co-occurring symptoms it is difficult to differentiate between disorders and the likelihood that a co-morbid disorder will be missed is increased. This emphasizes the need for assessment in multiple settings and reassessment over time.

One of the most compelling cross cultural descriptions of how autism is regarded across various cultures was the book *Unstrange Minds*. Written by the anthropologist Roy Grinker (2008), Grinker explains how the category of ASD is contingent on the culture through which it is expressed- the condition is associated with differing levels of stigma in different cultures. In the US, several studies have also shown that clinicians may diagnose ASD when resources are targeted at the diagnosis, whereas previously, under other circumstances, they may have diagnosed another category of childhood disorder. Paul Shattuck has written about the extent to which increases in the administrative prevalence of autism have been associated with corresponding decreases in the use of other diagnostic categories, mental retardation and learning disabilities (2006). This process of 'diagnostic substitution' he argues, may partially explain the rise in prevalence in autism in the US.

Our own work suggests that since the 1980s, the recorded prevalence of both ASD and ADHD in the UK has increased dramatically. We examined data from both the Millennium Cohort Study, (the large cohort of around 19,000 children who have been followed from their birth through to seven years old and beyond), and another cohort, called the British Cohort Study, where children were born thirty years previously. Both cohorts were representative of the UK as a whole, and medical reports of both ASD and ADHD were given when children were age seven for in 2007-9 and ten in 1980. The results from 2007 contrasted with the 1980 sample at age 10. Only 11 children in the 1970 British Cohort Study were reported as having ADHD in their medical exam, giving an estimated prevalence of 0.083%. The autism diagnosis was rarely used with just 3 children assigned the label; 0.023% of children. A number of other child psychiatric diagnoses were available and many of these were diagnosed during the medical exams. Details of these alternative labels are given in Table 1.

1980 Diagnosis (ICD 9 codes)	N of children	Percentage of total examined %
Autism (299.0/1/8/9)	3	0.023
ADHD (314.00/01, 314.9)	11	0.083
Disturbance in emotions (313)	7	0.053
Delays in development: Reading (315.0)	13	0.098
Delays in learning & development (315.2/8/9/5)	81	0.614
Delays in language (315.3)	62 (1 autism co-morbid)	0.462
Impulse control (312.3/9)	1	0.007
Mild mental retardation (317)	34 (1 ADHD co-morbid)	0.258
Other specified delays in development (318)	22 (1 ADHD co-morbid)	0.166

1980 Diagnosis (ICD 9 codes)	N of children	Percentage of total examined %
Unspecified delays in development (319)	25 (1 ADHD co-morbid)	0.379
Total	259	1.961

Table 1. Named conditions using ICD-9 categories for 10 year old children in 1980 (n=13201).

Among the 14,043 children in the 2007 cohort, 209 (1.49%) were reported to have ASD, and 180 (1.28%) were reported having been given an ADHD diagnosis by a clinician (unweighted figures). There was disproportional stratification in the Millennium Cohort, meaning that all analyses were weighted to account for the clustering and over-inclusion of participants from disadvantaged areas. After weighting, 1.7 % of children were reported as having an ASD (95% CI, 1.4-1.99). 1.3% of these were boys, and 0.25% girls, giving boy girl ratio of approx 5:1 for ASD. Surprisingly, the figure for ADHD was lower. After weighting, 1.4% of the population were reported as having ADHD (95% CI, 1.2-1.7). Of these, 2.3% were boys and 0.25% girls, giving a gender ratio of approximately of 1 girl to every 4 boys with ADHD.

One interpretation of the historical shift is that diagnostic substitution has occurred: children with similar symptoms in 1980 may have been more likely to receive generalised labels of 'delays in learning & development' than ASD or ADHD. So changing diagnostic practice, cultural factors and context may do much to explain both co-morbidity and rising prevalence. The steep rise in children assigned these diagnoses cannot be totally explained by the substitution mechanism- twice as many children were given either ASD or ADHD diagnoses in 2009 as the total number diagnosed with any type of developmental disorder in 1980.

Context also has a big part to play in the identification of difficulties, in terms of what is considered to be 'disordered'. Social constructionists have also pointed out that the conceptualization of difficulties associated with both dyslexia and ASD as 'disorders' is itself a product of social and cultural standards, and of course the definition of each disorder has changed over time. This has prompted calls for the term autism spectrum 'conditions' to replace autism spectrum 'disorders' (2009). Our own analysis of the Millennium Cohort has shown a strong association between ADHD and poverty, reflecting findings from US studies which have also found differing levels of ADHD amongst various ethnic groups- Hispanic children were more likely to be identified with ADHD in a study by Akinbami et al. (2011). It is unclear whether this is entirely due to greater awareness and access to health care in some groups, differential reporting about the same level of difficulties between ethnic groups or whether children in different groups have truly varying symptom levels (Boyle et al., 2011). A study by Cuccaro et al. (1996) showed the nature of diagnosis of developmental disorders varied according to the socio-economic status of the child's family; autism was more likely to be identified in children of higher income families, although no biases of SES were found for identification with ADHD. Cooper (2001) points out that the behaviour symptomatic of ADHD becomes problematic where high value is placed on ability to remain sedentary and sustain attention on tasks, in other words, in schools. Hulme and Snowling (2009) describe how differences of this nature must therefore be thought of as *both* biological *and* as a product of the social and environmental world.

12. Conclusion

Two conclusions can be drawn. First, co-morbidities between developmental disorders are common, and second, the causes of these overlapping difficulties are likely to be complex, multifactorial and interacting. Firstly, the high overlap between symptoms of different developmental disorders has been identified in a number of studies and there is an international consensus on this overlap. Studies from Canada, the UK, USA and Scandinavia all show how hard it is provide an unequivocal diagnosis, leading to the quote from Kaplan and her colleagues (2001) *in developmental disorders co-morbidity is the rule, not the exception*. This was informed by the group's work studying a population-based sample of 179 children receiving special support in Calgary: If the children met the dyslexia criteria, there was a 51.6% chance of having another disorder. If the children met the ADHD criteria there was an 80.4% chance of having another disorder. They criticize the term 'comorbidity', as it implies unsubstantiated presumption of independent aetiologies. The authors argue that discrete categories do not exist in real life.

Secondly, in considering the reasons for co-morbidities, a complex bio-psycho-social model is required that leads to symptoms that may result in diagnosis. The nature of the diagnosis itself may depend on social context as well as an individual child's behaviour. A hint of this complexity is achieved in Figure 3, which is a schematic diagram of various potential causal pathways. It is plausible that the same underlying genetic or neurological mechanisms may underlie co-occurrence of dyslexia, ADHD and ASD. The reverse pathways are not at first so obvious. But recent advances in systems biology have shown that the environment of the cell affects gene expression and protein synthesis at molecular levels. Thus environmental influences can alter 'core' biology: for example Mack and Mack (1992) describe how tweaking rats' whiskers changes gene expression in the sensory cortex. In systems theory, genetic influences are conceptualised more like a set of piano keys on which notes may be played or not played, played slowly or quickly, and there is enormous variation in the music produced even with the same basic set of keys. So the cellular environment can affect genetic expression. A simplified model underlying much behaviour genetics research envisages a direct linear relationship between individual genes and behaviours. The reality is likely to be far more complex with gene networks and multiple environmental factors impacting brain development and function, which in turn will influence behaviour (Hamer, 2002). Karmiloff-Smith (2007) emphasizes how learning and experience effects gene expression in humans. Such scholars demonstrate that the social can affect the biological as well as the more intuitive path of genetic origin leading to neurological development leading to aberrant behaviour. Diagnosis itself may influence behaviour too, through differential treatment and interventions. Thus the pervasive developmental environment is composed of many related factors, environmental stresses, and genetic predispositions, and the social contexts all of which may interact to produce developmental outcomes that themselves may contribute to predicting ongoing child development.

Snowling (2012) suggests a new dimensional classification of disorder, where deficits in different components of learning are seen as additive, impacting on the potential for remediation, rather than classing children into dichotomous 'disorder' categories. Taylor (2011) notes that for many children, it is better to think of changes in cognitive style, learning and motivation rather than symptoms. Both conclude that it is important to examine children for evidence of co-occurring disorders, and not simply continue to examine the areas which we expect to be impaired according to categorization. The practical application of assessing children for a range of difficulties is that children will be best helped not by any all encompassing diagnosis, but by individual analysis of their strengths and weaknesses. Future research may be wise to focus on the individual profiles of children across a broad range of areas, looking at the unique strengths, as well as the weaknesses of the individual children, so that parents and educators may adapt their support accordingly, regardless of the diagnostic label a child receives.

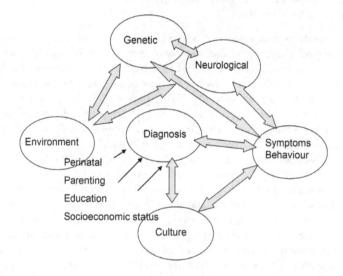

Figure 3. Schematic of interacting causal mechanisms for co-morbidity.

Author details

Ginny Russell[1] and Zsuzsa Pavelka[2]

1 University of Exeter Medical School, ESRC Centre for Genomics in Society, UK

2 University of Milan, Italy

References

[1] Akinbami, L. J., Liu, X., Pastor, P. N., & Reuben, C. A. (2011). Attention deficit hyper-activity disorder among children aged 5-17 years in the United States, 1998-2009. *NCHS Data Brief*, (70), 1–8.

[2] American Psychiatric Association. (2000). *Diagnostic and Statistical Manual of Mental Disorders* (4th ed., text revision [DSM-IV-TR]

[3] Bailey, A., & Parr, J. (2003). Implications of the broader phenotype for concepts of autism. *Novartis Foundation symposium, 251*, 26–35; discussion 36–47, 109–11, 281–97.

[4] Barkley, R. A. (2012). *Executive Functions: What They Are, How They Work, and Why They Evolved* (1st ed.). Guilford Press.

[5] Baron-Cohen, S, Leslie, A. M., & Frith, U. (1985). Does the autistic child have a 'theo-ry of mind'? *Cognition, 21*(1), 37–46.

[6] Baron-Cohen, Simon. (2002). The extreme male brain theory of autism. *Trends Cogn Sci, 6*(6), 248–254.

[7] Baron-Cohen, Simon, Scott, F. J., Allison, C., Williams, J., Bolton, P., Matthews, F. E., & Brayne, C. (2009). Prevalence of autism-spectrum conditions: UK school-based population study. *The British Journal of Psychiatry, 194*(6), 500–509.

[8] Bental, B., & Tirosh, E. (2007). The relationship between attention, executive func-tions and reading domain abilities in attention deficit hyperactivity disorder and reading disorder: A comparative study. *Journal of Child Psychology and Psychiatry, 48*(5), 455–463.

[9] Bolton, P. F., Murphy, M., Macdonald, H., Whitlock, B., Pickles, A., & Rutter, M. (1997). Obstetric complications in autism: consequences or causes of the condition? *Journal of the American Academy of Child and Adolescent Psychiatry, 36*(2), 272–81.

[10] Boyle, C. A., Boulet, S., Schieve, L. A., Cohen, R. A., Blumberg, S. J., Yeargin-Allsopp, M., Visser, S., et al. (2011). Trends in the prevalence of developmental disabilities in US children, 1997-2008. *Pediatrics, 127*(6), 1034–1042.

[11] Bradley, E. A., Summers, J. A., Wood, H. L., & Bryson, S. E. (2004). Comparing rates of psychiatric and behavior disorders in adolescents and young adults with severe intellectual disability with and without autism. *Journal of Autism and Developmental Disorders, 34*(2), 151–61.

[12] Bramham, J., Ambery, F., Young, S., Morris, R., Russell, A., Xenitidis, K., Asherson, P., et al. (2009). Executive functioning differences between adults with attention defi-cit hyperactivity disorder and autistic spectrum disorder in initiation, planning and strategy formation. *Autism, 13*(3), 245–264.

[13] British Psychological Society. (1999). Working party of the division of educational and child psychology of the British Psychological Society: Dyslexia, literacy and psychological assessment. *British Psychological Society* : Leicester.

[14] Cheslack-Postava, K., & Jordan-Young, R. M. (2012). Autism spectrum disorders: Toward a gendered embodiment model. *Social Science & Medicine (1982), 74*(11), 1667–1674.

[15] Cheung, C. H. M., Wood, A. C., Paloyelis, Y., Arias-Vasquez, A., Buitelaar, J. K., Franke, B., Miranda, A., et al. (2012). Aetiology for the covariation between combined type ADHD and reading difficulties in a family study: The role of IQ. *Journal of Child Psychology and Psychiatry,, 53*(8), 864–873.

[16] Clark, T., Feehan, C., Tinline, C., & Vostanis, P. (1999). Autistic symptoms in children with attention deficit-hyperactivity disorder. *European Child & Adolescent Psychiatry, 8*(1), 50–55.

[17] Coltheart, M., & Jackson, N. E. (1998). Defining Dyslexia. *Child and Adolescent Mental Health, 3*(1), 12–16.

[18] Constantino, J. N., & Todd, R. D. (2003). Autistic traits in the general population: A twin study. *Archives of general psychiatry, 60*(5), 524–30.

[19] Cooper, P. (2001). Understanding ADHD: A brief critical review of literature. *Children & Society, 15*(5), 387–95.

[20] Cuccaro, M. L., Wright, H. H., Rownd, C. V., Abramson, R. K., Waller, J., & Fender, D. (1996). Professional perceptions of children with developmental difficulties: The influence of race and socioeconomic status. *Journal of Autism and Developmental Disorders, 26*(4), 461–469.

[21] Daniels, J. L., Forssen, U., Hultman, C. M., Cnattingius, S., Savitz, D. A., Feychting, M., & Sparen, P. (2008). Parental psychiatric disorders associated with autism spectrum disorders in the offspring. *Pediatrics, 121*(5), e1357–1362.

[22] Danielsson, S., Gillberg, I. C., Billstedt, E., Gillberg, C., & Olsson, I. (2005). Epilepsy in young adults with autism: a prospective population-based follow-up study of 120 individuals diagnosed in childhood. *Epilepsia, 46*(6), 918–23.

[23] Deykin, E. Y., & MacMahon, B. (1980). Pregnancy, delivery, and neonatal complications among autistic children. *American Journal of Diseases of Children, 134*(9), 860-864.

[24] Dulcan, M. (1997). Practice parameters for the assessment and treatment of children, adolescents, and adults with attention-deficit/hyperactivity disorder. *Journal of the American Academy of Child and Adolescent Psychiatry, 36*(10 Suppl), 85S–121S.

[25] Elia, J., Ambrosini, P. J., & Rapoport, J. L. (1999). Treatment of attention-deficit–hyperactivity disorder. *New England Journal of Medicine, 340*(10), 780–788.

[26] Ericson, R. V., & Doyle, A. (2003). *Risk and Morality*. University of Toronto Press.

[27] Evans, D. W., Canavera, K., Kleinpeter, F. L., Maccubbin, E., & Taga, K. (2005). The fears, phobias and anxieties of children with autism spectrum disorders and Down syndrome: Comparisons with developmentally and chronologically age matched children. *Child Psychiatry and Human Development, 36*(1), 3–26.

[28] Fawcett, A. (2012). Introduction to Dyslexia and Co-occuring Difficulties. *Dylexia and co-occuring difficulties*. Bracknell, UK: British Dyslexia Association.

[29] Felicetti, T. (1981). Parents of autistic children: Some notes on a chemical connection. *Milieu Therapy, 1*, 13–16.

[30] Freitag, C. M. (2007). The genetics of autistic disorders and its clinical relevance: A review of the literature. *Molecular Psychiatry, 12*(1), 2–22.

[31] Frith, U. (2003). *Autism: Explaining the Enigma* (2nd Ed.). Oxford, UK: Wiley-Black-well.

[32] Frith, U., & Happé, F. (1998). Why specific developmental disorders are not specific: On-line and developmental effects in autism and dyslexia. *Developmental Science, 1*(2), 267–272.

[33] Gillberg, C. (2010). The ESSENCE in child psychiatry: Early Symptomatic Syndromes Eliciting Neurodevelopmental Clinical Examinations. *Research in developmental disabilities, 31*(6), 1543–1551.

[34] Gooch, D., Snowling, M., & Hulme, C. (2011). Time perception, phonological skills and executive function in children with dyslexia and/or ADHD symptoms. *Journal of Child Psychology and Psychiatry, 52*(2), 195–203.

[35] Goodman, R., & Scott, S. (1997). *Child Psychiatry*. (2nd ed.). Oxford, UK: Blackwell Publishing.

[36] Griffiths, C. C. B. (2007). Pragmatic abilities in adults with and without dyslexia: A pilot study. *Dyslexia, 13*(4), 276–296.

[37] Grinker, R. R. (2008). *Unstrange minds: Remapping the world of autism*. Cambridge, MA: Basic Books.

[38] Hamer, D. (2002). Genetics: Rethinking behavior genetics. *Science, 298*(5591), 71–72.

[39] Happé, F. G. (1994). Current psychological theories of autism: The 'theory of mind' account and rival theories. *Journal of Child Psychology and Psychiatry, 35*(2), 215–29.

[40] Happé, F., Ronald, A., & Plomin, R. (2006). Time to give up on a single explanation for autism. *Nature Neuroscience, 9*, 1218–1220.

[41] Happé, Francesca, & Frith, U. (2006). The weak coherence account: detail-focused cognitive style in autism spectrum disorders. *Journal of Autism and Developmental Disorders, 36*(1), 5–25.

[42] Hedgecoe, A. (2001). Schizophrenia and the narrative of enlightened geneticization. *Social Studies of Science, 31*(6), 875–911.

[43] Hill, E. L. (2004). Executive dysfunction in autism. *Trends in Cognitive Sciences, 8*(1), 26–32.

[44] Hofvander, B., Delorme, R., Chaste, P., Nydén, A., Wentz, E., Ståhlberg, O., Herbrecht, E., et al. (2009). Psychiatric and psychosocial problems in adults with normal-intelligence autism spectrum disorders. *BMC Psychiatry, 9,* 35.

[45] Howlin, P. (2000). Outcome in adult life for more able individuals with autism or Asperger syndrome. *Autism, 4*(1), 63–83.

[46] Hulme, C., & Snowling, M. J. (2009). *Developmental disorders of language learning and cognition.* Chichester, UK: Wiley-Blackwell.

[47] Iacoboni, M., & Dapretto, M. (2006). The mirror neuron system and the consequences of its dysfunction. *Nature reviews. Neuroscience, 7*(12), 942–51.

[48] Ingudomnukul, E., Baron-Cohen, S., Wheelwright, S., & Knickmeyer, R. (2007). Elevated rates of testosterone-related disorders in women with autism spectrum conditions. *Hormones and Behavior, 51*(5), 597–604.

[49] Kadesjö, B., Gillberg, C., & Hagberg, B. (1999). Brief Report: Autism and Asperger syndrome in seven-year-old children: A total population study. *Journal of Autism and Developmental Disorders, 29*(4), 327–331.

[50] Kaplan, B. J., Dewey, D. M., Crawford, S. G., & Wilson, B. N. (2001). The term comorbidity is of questionable value in reference to developmental disorders: Data and theory. *Journal of Learning Disabilities, 34*(6), 555–565.

[51] Karmiloff-Smith, A. (2007). Atypical epigenesis. *Developmental Science, 10*(1), 84–88.

[52] Kessler, R. C., Adler, L., Ames, M., Demler, O., Faraone, S., Hiripi, E., Howes, M. J., et al. (2005). The World Health Organization adult ADHD self-report scale (ASRS): a short screening scale for use in the general population. *Psychological Medicine, 35*(2), 245–256.

[53] Kielinen, M., Rantala, H., Timonen, E., Linna, S.-L., & Moilanen, I. (2004). Associated medical disorders and disabilities in children with autistic disorder: A population-based study. *Autism, 8*(1), 49–60.

[54] Kolevzon, A., Gross, R., & Reichenberg, A. (2007). Prenatal and perinatal risk factors for autism: A review and integration of findings. *Archives of Pediatrics & Adolescent Medicine, 161*(4), 326–33.

[55] London, E. (2007). The role of the neurobiologist in redefining the diagnosis of autism. *Brain pathology (Zurich, Switzerland), 17*(4), 408–11.

[56] Mack, K. J., & Mack, P. A. (1992). Induction of transcription factors in somatosensory cortex after tactile stimulation. *Molecular Brain Research, 12*(1-3), 141–147.

[57] Miles, T. R. (2004). Some problems in determining the prevalence of dyslexia. *Electronic Journal of Research in Educational Psychology, 2*(2), 5–12.

[58] Mulligan, A., Anney, R. J. L., O'Regan, M., Chen, W., Butler, L., Fitzgerald, M., Buitelaar, J., et al. (2009). Autism symptoms in Attention-Deficit/Hyperactivity Disorder:
A familial trait which correlates with conduct, oppositional defiant, language and
motor disorders. *Journal of Autism and Developmental Disorders, 39*(2), 197–209.

[59] Mulligan, A., Anney, R., Butler, L., O'Regan, M., Richardson, T., Tulewicz, E. M.,
Fitzgerald, M. Gill, M. (2011). Home environment: association with hyperactivity impulsivity in children with ADHD and their non-ADHD siblings. *Child: Care, Health
and Development* [e-pub ahead of print].

[60] Newschaffer, C. J., Croen, L. A., Daniels, J., Giarelli, E., Grether, J. K., Levy, S. E.,
Mandell, D. S., Miller, L.A., Pinto-Martin, J, Reaven, J., Reynolds, A.M., Rice, C.E.,
Schendel, D., Windham, G.C.(2007). The epidemiology of autism spectrum disorders.
Annual Review of Public Health, 28, 235-58.

[61] Nydén, A., Gillberg, C., Hjelmquist, E., & Heiman, M. (1999). Executive function/
attention deficits in boys with Asperger syndrome, attention disorder and reading/
writing disorder. *Autism, 3*(3), 213–228.

[62] Posserud, M.-B., Lundervold, A. J., & Gillberg, C. (2006). Autistic features in a total
population of 7-9-year-old children assessed by the ASSQ (Autism Spectrum Screening Questionnaire). *Journal of Child Psychology and Psychiatry, 47*(2), 167–75.

[63] Reiersen, A. M., Constantino, J. N., Grimmer, M., Martin, N. G., & Todd, R. D. (2008).
Evidence for shared genetic influences on self-reported ADHD and autistic symptoms in young adult Australian twins. *Twin Research and Human Genetics, 11*(6), 579–
585.

[64] Reiersen, Angela M, & Todd, R. D. (2008). Co-occurrence of ADHD and autism spectrum disorders: phenomenology and treatment. *Expert Review of Neurotherapeutics,
8*(4), 657–669.

[65] Richardson, A. J. (2006). Omega-3 fatty acids in ADHD and related neurodevelopmental disorders. *International Review of Psychiatry, 18*(2), 155–172.

[66] Ronald, A., Edelson, L. R., Asherson, P., & Saudino, K. J. (2010). Exploring the relationship between autistic-like traits and ADHD behaviors in early childhood: Findings from a community twin study of 2-year-olds. *Journal of Abnormal Child
Psychology, 38*(2), 185–196.

[67] Russell, G., Golding, J., Norwich, B., Emond, A., Ford, T., & Steer, C. (2012). Social
and behavioural outcomes in children diagnosed with autism spectrum disorders: A
longitudinal cohort study. *Journal of Child Psychology and Psychiatry, 53*(7), 735–744.

[68] Russell, G., & Kelly, S. (2011). Looking beyond risk: A study of lay epidemiology of
childhood disorders. *Health, Risk & Society, 13*(2), 129.

[69] Russell, G., Norwich, B., & Gwernan-Jones, R. (2012). When diagnosis is uncertain:
variation in conclusions after psychological assessment of a six-year-old child. *Early
Child Development and Care*, (early on-line version).

[70] Russell, G., Steer, C., & Golding, J. (2011). Social and demographic factors that influ-
      ence the diagnosis of autistic spectrum disorders. *Social Psychiatry and Psychiatric Epi-
      demiology, 46*(12), 1283–1293.

[71] Rutter, M. (2005). Incidence of autism spectrum disorders: changes over time and
      their meaning. *Acta paediatrica, 94*(1), 2–15.

[72] Rutter, M., Andersen-Wood, L., Beckett, C., Bredenkamp, D., Castle, J., Groothues,
      C., Kreppner, J., et al. (1999). Quasi-autistic patterns following severe early global
      privation. English and Romanian Adoptees (ERA) Study Team. *Journal of Child Psy-
      chology and Psychiatry, , 40*(4), 537–549.

[73] Sanders, S. J., Murtha, M. T., Gupta, A. R., Murdoch, J. D., Raubeson, M. J., Willsey,
      A. J., Ercan-Sencicek, A. G., et al. (2012). De novo mutations revealed by whole-
      exome sequencing are strongly associated with autism. *Nature.*

[74] Santosh, P. J., & Mijovic, A. (2004). Social impairment in hyperkinetic disorder - rela-
      tionship to psychopathology and environmental stressors. *European Child & Adoles-
      cent Psychiatry, 13*(3), 141–150.

[75] Sciutto, M. J., Nolfi, C. J., & Bluhm, C. (2004). Effects of child gender and symptom
      type on referrals for ADHD by elementary school teachers. *Journal of Emotional and
      Behavioral Disorders, 12*(4), 247–253.

[76] Shattuck, P. T. (2006). The contribution of diagnostic substitution to the growing ad-
      ministrative prevalence of autism in US special education. *Pediatrics, 117*(4), 1028–37.

[77] Simonoff, E., Pickles, A., Charman, T., Chandler, S., Loucas, T., & Baird, G. (2008).
      Psychiatric disorders in children with autism spectrum disorders: prevalence, comor-
      bidity, and associated factors in a population-derived sample. *Journal of the American
      Academy of Child and Adolescent Psychiatry, 47*(8), 921–929.

[78] Snowling, M. J. (2012). Editorial: Seeking a new characterisation of learning disor-
      ders. *Journal of Child Psychology and Psychiatry 53*(1), 1–2.

[79] Sonuga-Barke, E. J. S., & Halperin, J. M. (2010). Developmental phenotypes and caus-
      al pathways in attention deficit/hyperactivity disorder: Potential targets for early in-
      tervention? *Journal of Child Psychology and Psychiatry, 51*(4), 368–389.

[80] Sturm, H., Fernell, E., & Gillberg, C. (2004). Autism spectrum disorders in children
      with normal intellectual levels: Associated impairments and subgroups. *Developmen-
      tal Medicine and Child Neurology, 46*(7), 444–7.

[81] Taylor, E. (2011). Commentary: Reading and attention problems – how are they con-
      nected? Reflections on reading McGrath et al. (2011). *Journal of Child Psychology and
      Psychiatry, 52*(5), 558–559.

[82] Trottier, G., Srivastava, L., & Walker, C. D. (1999). Etiology of infantile autism: A re-
      view of recent advances in genetic and neurobiological research. *Journal of Psychiatry
      and Neuroscience, 24*(2), 103-15.

[83] Turner, M. (1999). Annotation: Repetitive behaviour in autism: A review of psychological research. *Journal of Child Psychology and Psychiatry, 40*(6), 839–849.

[84] Willcutt, E. G., Doyle, A. E., Nigg, J. T., Faraone, S. V., & Pennington, B. F. (2005).
Validity of the executive function theory of attention-deficit/hyperactivity disorder:
A meta-analytic review. *Biological Psychiatry, 57*(11), 1336–1346.

[85] Williams, D. (1992). *Nobody nowhere: The extraordinary autobiography of an autistic* (1st
ed.). New York, NY: HarperCollins.

[86] World Health Organization. (1992). *International Classification of Diseases and related
health problems (ICD-10).* Geneva, WHO. Retrieved from www.who.int/
classifications/icd/en/greenbook.pdf p.179

[87] Wright, C., Conlon, E., Wright, M., & Dyck, M. (2011). Sub-lexical reading intervention in a student with dyslexia and Asperger's disorder. *Australian Journal of Educational & Developmental Psychology, 11*, 11–25.

[88] Zwaigenbaum, L., Szatmari, P., Jones, M. B., Bryson, S. E., MacLean, J. E., Mahoney,
W. J., Bartolucci, G., et al. (2002). Pregnancy and birth complications in autism and
liability to the broader autism phenotype. *Journal of the American Academy of Child and
Adolescent Psychiatry, 41*(5), 572–9.

Aetiological Factors - Sensory Issues, Foetal Alcohol Syndrome and Relationships

Chapter 3

Relationships, Sexuality, and Intimacy in Autism Spectrum Disorders

Maria R. Urbano, Kathrin Hartmann,
Stephen I. Deutsch,
Gina M. Bondi Polychronopoulos and
Vanessa Dorbin

Additional information is available at the end of the chapter

1. Introduction

The purpose of this chapter is to provide a brief overview of Autism Spectrum Disorders (ASD) and sexuality, as there is a paucity of this information in the literature. Specific attention is given to sexuality involving the self, others, and interpersonal relationships. Problematic sexual behaviors, legal concerns, and sexual abuse (including victimization and perpetration) are also discussed. Finally, intervention strategies for ASD children, adults, and families are addressed. The overall aim of this chapter is to highlight major themes regarding Autism Spectrum Disorders and sexuality while contributing to the existing literature.

2. Autism overview

Autism Spectrum Disorders, as currently defined by the Diagnostic and Statistical Manual (DSM-IV-TR) criteria, include the diagnoses of Autistic Disorder, Asperger's Disorder and Pervasive Developmental Disorder NOS. The three major diagnostic categories include the following: 1) language impairment, 2) social impairment, and 3) repetitive behaviors/restricted interests, with the impairments present prior to the age of three. Autism has been conceptualized under this diagnostic rubric as a spectrum of disorders with symptoms ranging from severe to minimally impaired [1]. With the advent of the DSM-5, only two major criteria will be included: 1) social communication impairment, and 2) repetitive behaviors/restricted interests.

The DSM-5 envisions autism as a unitary diagnosis with multiple levels of symptom severity impairing the ability to function [2]. The DSM-5 will use a system of three modifiers to signify level of severity: Level 1 is characterized for patients requiring support as they display difficulty initiating social situations and demonstrate atypical social responses. Rituals and repetitive behaviors cause significant interference for these individuals. They also resist redirection and attempts to be interrupted when involved in restricted interests or repetitive behaviors. Level 2 is characterized for patients "requiring substantial support," as they have marked deficits in verbal and nonverbal social communication skills, which are apparent even with supports in place. They demonstrate limited ability to initiate social interaction and have a reduced or abnormal response to social overtures from others. Repetitive behaviors and restricted interests are obvious enough to be noticed by a casual observer. These patients become distressed or frustrated when they are interrupted or redirected. Level 3 is characterized for patients requiring very substantial support, as they have severe deficits in verbal and nonverbal social communication skills. Repetitive behaviors or rituals markedly interfere with functioning in all spheres. They demonstrate marked distress when routines are interrupted, and they are very difficult to redirect [2].

Proposed changes to the DSM-5 diagnostic criteria include the creation of a single broad autism spectrum disorder (ASD) diagnosis that encompasses current specific DSM-IV-TR diagnoses. Further, the proposed DSM-5 criteria reflect the tension between considering core symptoms from a dimensional perspective (i.e., symptoms are distributed in the population and patients are distinguished from unaffected persons by the severity of their symptoms), as opposed to the presence of discrete symptoms reflecting categorical distinctions between affected and unaffected persons [3]. A dimensional approach suggests that the core symptoms are quantitative traits which vary along a continuum and reflect the expression of, and interactions between, commonly occurring genetic variations and effects of environmental factors, whereas categorical approaches favor models attributing risk of illness to large effects of single genes, especially genes involved in brain development or maintenance of synaptic architecture [3]. In fact, the DSM-5 diagnostic criteria may be best represented by an empirically-derived hybrid model that merges the dimensional and categorical aspects of symptoms of autism (i.e., there are threshold values for numbers and severity of symptoms that define a categorical diagnosis of an ASD). From a biological perspective, although symptoms may be viewed along a continuum, the diagnosis of autism implies the altered, albeit subtle, architecture of the brain. The two core symptom domains of DSM-5, whose severity can vary along a continuum, were validated independently and include 1) impaired social communication and interaction (SCI), and 2) restricted, repetitive behavior (RRB) [3,4]. There is still work left to be done with respect to determining the number of criteria that must be satisfied in order to assign an ASD diagnosis. The DSM-5 criteria are clearly being shown as superior to the DSM-IV-TR criteria in terms of specificity. However, a balance must be struck between reducing "false positives," which maximizes specificity, and assuring that criteria are sufficiently sensitive to capture ASD-affected persons that would benefit from intervention and services. This is an especially big concern among caregivers of persons that would have previously received a diagnosis of Asperger's disorder and for children and adolescents with poor historical information about early-life symptoms (e.g., children and youth in foster and juvenile justice settings). Inclusion of "subtler" symptoms, such as those reflected in the following items from the Social Responsiveness Scale (© Western Psychological Services), improved the sensitivity of identifying persons with high-functioning ASD (such as persons diagnosed with Asperger's disorder): impaired social understanding or awareness, literal or pedantic use of language, difficulties in adjusting behavior to various contexts, unusual prosody, and problems with body orientation or social distance [3]. Additional research must be conducted to determine the discriminative diagnostic value should be placed [4].

Along with the proposed diagnostic criteria, estimates of the prevalence of autism have also changed. Recently, the prevalence estimates of the Autism and Developmental Disabilities Monitoring (ADDM) Network for children aged 8 years utilized a consistent "records-based" surveillance methodology in 14 sites across the United States, examining both health and education records [5]. The overall estimated 2008 prevalence of autism spectrum disorders was 1 in 88 children, demonstrating a steady increase in prevalence since 2002 [6]. Although the ADDM Network sites are not a nationally representative sample, the methodology used in obtaining prevalence estimates of children aged 8 years has been consistent since the monitoring began, so valid comparisons can be made with earlier years. These comparisons show that the estimated prevalence in 2008 increased by 23% in comparison to 2006, and by 78% when compared to 2002. The increase in prevalence may simply reflect greater awareness and better ascertainment of autism spectrum disorders by health agencies and schools, as suggested in a community mental health surveillance study in England [7]. The England study showed that the prevalence of autism in adults, when properly diagnosed, was approximately the same as in children.

3. Normal sexual development

Sexual development is a complex process that includes sexuality in relation to oneself and others. Sexuality encompasses a broad variety of physical, emotional, and social interactions. It includes sexual beliefs, attitudes, knowledge, values, and behavior and concerns the anatomy, physiology, and biochemistry of the sexual response system. Sexuality involves one's thoughts, feelings, behaviors, relationships, roles, identity, and personality [8].

As with other individuals, those with ASD grow and mature along many developmental lines [9]. The social developmental line includes the development of sexuality, while the physical line includes that of puberty. Sexuality begins in infancy and progresses through adulthood until death. Each life stage brings about physical changes and psychosocial demands that need to be achieved for sexual health to be attained. The capacity for a sexual response, both male and female, has been found as early as in the 24-hour period after birth. The rhythmic manipulation of genitals similar to adult masturbation begins at 2.5 to 3 years of age are a natural form of sexual expression [10]. Also during the first three years of life, a child forms an attachment to his or her parents that is facilitated by physical contact. A stable, secure attachment with parents enhances the possibility of such an attachment when an adult is preparing to meet an intimate partner [10]. Gender identity, i.e. one's sense of male-ness or femaleness, also forms in the first three years of life. A clear, secure gender identity allows for satisfying, intimate adult relationships. Children may display masturbatory be-haviors and engage in a variety of sexual play activities that coincide with the development of socially expected norms in the context of natural curiosity about themselves and their en-vironment. Between the ages of 3 to 7, children explore their own body parts, recognize them as male or female, and become interested in the genitals of their peers, leading to sexu-al play [10]. During the latency years, overt sexual play becomes covert, with children begin-ning to have experience with masturbation, should libidinal urges occur. As latency-age children segregate along sexual lines, any sexual experiences are usually with those of the same gender [10]. More overt behaviors and interests emerge again in adolescence with the onset of puberty. Reports collected by the Centers for Disease Control and Prevention (CDC) in 2000 showed about 52% of males and 48% of females in grades 9 to 12 are engaging in sexual intercourse as reported by Delamater and Friedrich in 2002 [10]. Similar statistics were reported as recently as 2011 by the CDC, with 47.4% of 9-12th graders reporting that they had ever engaged in sexual intercourse [11]. Cultural differences are also apparent among groups regarding premarital intercourse [10].

Pubertal changes can begin as early as 9 years of age or as late as 14 years of age. With the onset of puberty, sexual development moves to the forefront. Puberty, governed by hormo-nal changes, is defined as the time when a male or female is capable of sexual reproduction. A growth spurt, skeletal changes, increases in muscle and fat tissue, development of breasts, pubic and axillary hair, and the growth of genitalia are all hallmarks of the pubertal process [12]. With the physical maturation of gonads, genitalia and secondary sex characteristics, one's sexual interest increases. Citing a study by Bancroft and colleagues (2003), Delamater and Friedrich noted that many males begin to masturbate between the ages of 13 and 15, whereas the onset for girls is more varied [10]. As older adolescents and young adults devel-op, more teens engage in sexual intercourse and develop a sexually active heterosexual life-style. Between 5 and 10% of adolescent males, and 6% of adolescent females, experiment with homosexual behavior. This exploration may be a transient experience, or it may devel-op into an adult homosexual identity [10]. One of the major psychological developmental tasks of later adolescence is to develop a firm sense of identity, of which one's gender identi-ty is an important aspect [13]. Achieving sexual maturity continues into adulthood with the ability to make informed decisions about one's partner choice, reproduction, and long-term intimate relationships.

4. Sexuality, disability, and ASD

Sexual development is an intricate process that examines sexuality in regard to oneself and others. This process is often thought of in terms of normal development; however the devel-opmentally disabled also go through sexual stages as they physically mature. This concept can be difficult to accept for some providers and caretakers, due to their tendency to view the developmentally disabled as perennial children [14].

For much of our history, the concept that individuals with any disability as sexual beings was unthinkable [15]. Those with developmental disabilities were frequently subjected to involuntary sterilization in the first half of the 20th century. The sexual nature of those with disabilities has been traditionally denied and/or ignored. It has also been viewed similarly with ASD individuals, whose sexuality is further complicated by social communication and language deficits [15]. Only recently has it been acknowledged that persons with ASD have the universal right to learn about relationships, marriage, parenthood, and appropriate sexuality [8]. A major contribution to the field of autism and sexuality is the TEACCH Report published through the United Kingdom [16]. This article, based on the approach and concepts developed by Mesibov and Schopler [17] in the 1980's, put forth five basic assumptions concerning those with autism and are quoted below.

1.   People with autism of all levels of severity experience sexual drives, behaviors, or feelings with which at some point in their lives they need assistance

2.   Parent involvement and participation is a crucial ingredient in the area of sexual education

3.   Sexual education must be taught in a highly structured, individualized way using concrete strategies with less of an emotional overtone

4.   Sexual behaviors must be an important behavioral priority with less tolerance for deviations in this area due to the stringent expectations of society

5.   Sexual education must be taught in a specific individualized, developmental manner [16]

This report was one of the first to acknowledge that individuals with autism have the same human sexual urges and behaviors as all humans and that those with ASD have the right to express their sexuality to the greatest level possible. These tenets therefore emphasize the need for sexual education for those with ASD, so they can be integrated into our society's rules concerning what sexual behaviors are considered either appropriate or inappropriate.

Keeping in mind that quite often individuals with ASD may also have an intellectual disability [18], studies of individuals with a disability in general become important for the ASD population as well. The current literature already being conducted for those with disabilities is being applied to the expressed needs for education of those with ASD on how to develop sexual and intimate relationships. One study identified that those under the age of 18 had only limited knowledge about pregnancy and sexual anatomy while most individuals including adults were aspiring to form relationships and marriage [19]. In addition, general reluctance of family members and caregivers to acknowledge and respect the sexual rights of those with an intellectual disability was identified because these concepts created a certain level of anxiety in those family members.

As with others individuals who have a disability, those with an Autism Spectrum Disorder diagnosis possess the right to have a relationship, to marry, and/or to have children. Education about legal rights should be provided to those with ASD and extended especially to those whom they encounter, e.g. teachers, family, policemen, community members, etc. Education and awareness are key factors in the ability to identify violations to individuals' basic human rights.

Although those with an ASD diagnosis have the right to date, marry and have children, there is a paucity of empirical research on family units and relationships for this particular group. Though some evidence does exist anecdotally, e.g. through blogs and books, this evidence is not scientifically sound. Therefore, future research should generate empirical studies that focus on interpersonal relationships within the family unit and examine which factors or skills may contribute to their success.

5. Characteristics common to ASD persons

The overarching confounding factor for individuals with ASD to develop normative sexual identity, sexual orientation, and sexual behaviors is their core social disability [20] that in turn influences the person's opportunity and availability for romantic and intimate relationships. While levels of romantic and sexual functioning typically increase with age, a developmental lag was reported for individuals with ASD [21]. In a survey of parents of 38 neurotypically developing adolescents and young adults and 25 adolescents and young adults with ASD, Stokes and colleagues found support for their research hypotheses that individuals with ASD had less access to peers and friends, engaged in more unacceptable behaviors in attempting to initiate romantic relationships, and persisted in their pursuit of the relationship even when non-mutual interests were evident [21]. In 2012, Shandra and Chowdhury conducted a study on the first sexual experiences of adolescent girls with and without disabilities and reported that social isolation (not the adolescents' impairment) was the primary contributor to difficulties, based on their review of the literature and analyses of a national longitudinal data bank. Results also suggested that having a mild disability increased the likelihood of having sexual intercourse with a stranger for the first time, rather than with a steady dating partner [22].

Several characteristics of those with ASD interfere with the capacity to develop meaningful adult social relationships, which are necessary for developing sexual, intimate relationships. Foremost is the difficulty with social judgment [8], i.e. missing nonverbal communication, poor eye contact, theory of mind problems, and flexibility in response. Lack of experience in peer relationships prevents the development of the common pathway through which adolescents learn about sexuality [23]. Problematic decision-making skills complicate the capacity to maintain the everyday details of a relationship, such as initiating dates, or remembering plans. Lack of flexibility, along with self-absorption, creates significant areas of conflict in a potential relationship. Emotional dysregulation resulting in feelings that are too intense, or perhaps misplaced, together with a lack of awareness of the other's response can quickly end a relationship. Sensory sensitivities, such as inability to tolerate touch or other physical sensations, sound sensitivities, or food texture issues can cause dating to be fraught with problems [24].

Many persons with ASD have little self-awareness and as noted above, do not understand their impact on others. Another dimension of this issue is that persons with ASD may have little knowledge about themselves. Part of what helps us create a sense of self is the ability to create an internal autobiography [25]. Persons with ASD have difficulty in this area, as they frequently cannot describe their own emotions or are unaware of what they are feeling (i.e. alexithymia) or have difficulty controlling their emotional responses (i.e. emotion dysregulation). As a result, many with ASD lack the ability to insightfully understand themselves or respond to the social climate in a meaningful way. Self-advocacy, a crucial skill for maintaining one's function in daily life, is something that can be very difficult for a person with ASD to learn. The ability to maintain personal safety without awareness of the environment or the behaviors of others can pose a significant danger.

Persons with ASD, either as a result of the above difficulties or due to a true lack of social interest, turn away from others into their own world. Self-absorption fosters another type of social disability. Persons with ASD frequently have restricted areas of interest (e.g. computer animation) and may have little to no desire in sharing this interest with others or attending to the interests of others, since there can be a lack of ability to detach from the area of interest without anxiety or distress. The need for sameness and rigidity in daily routines may supersede one's ability to flexibly respond to another person, e.g. being unable to eat at another restaurant when only two specific restaurants are in that person's repertoire [26]. The need for aloneness or "down time" may be greater than the need to be with others, which may seriously jeopardize an attempt to relate to others in a more than superficial manner. Sensory sensitivities can create intolerance of what may be considered part of the human experience. For example, sensitivity to sound may prevent a person with ASD from engaging in activities where airplanes may be heard overhead or babies may be heard crying. Also, sensitivity to touch can be especially difficult in relation to others, as those with ASD may not tolerate someone touching their skin or attempting to hug them. This particular sensitivity may also affect the choice of clothes for someone with ASD, who may be unable to wear clothes with sleeves or tags that they feel are restrictive and might lead one to wear socially inappropriate apparel.

Executive function impairments, i.e. impairments in decision-making skills, cognitive flexibility, impulse control, organizational skills, and planning, create another layer of social dysfunction [27]. Awareness of the passage of time may be compromised for someone with ASD, perhaps secondary to their self-absorption, and is an essential component of everyday function. Everyday memory problems or the ability to remember to plan and organize daily life activities can create social havoc. The ability to problem solve, make informed choices, or plan for the future becomes problematic in what is called "context blindness" [27].

All of the above challenges are magnified when a person with ASD attempts to have an intimate emotional and perhaps sexual relationship. Intimacy is the sharing of emotional, cognitive, and physical aspects of oneself with those of another. A prerequisite for intimacy is the establishment of a firm sense of self-identity. Intimacy requires the flexibility to loosen one's identity in order to feel the pleasure of merging with one's partner in an emotional and physical connection. For all of the reasons above, a person with ASD may be unable to share with another or may be limited in his or her ability to do so.

Case example: RJ

RJ is a 28 year-old female with ASD who was attempting to negotiate an intimate relationship with another woman her age that did not have ASD. First of all, RJ explained that a homosexual relationship was better for her than a heterosexual relationship because her partner was more like her than another man would be, and it was already very difficult to consider an intimate relationship, let alone try to understand someone of a different gender. RJ was absorbed in her interest in drawing and hoped to get a job at some point in computer animation. She spent most of the hours in a day drawing when she was not at her part time job at the local animal shelter. When she was drawing, it was fine for her partner to sit next to her, but she didn't want to be disturbed or touched. She was unable to do something other than drawing in the evening except on Saturdays, when she was able to include her partner in her schedule. Even on Saturday, she needed to find some time to herself because it took too much energy to be with her partner for a full day. When she attempted to do so, she would experience anxiety and frustration which would frequently culminate in an episode of yelling, stamping her feet, and retreating to her room. On Saturdays, when she was attempting to spend time with her partner, RJ was only able to engage in certain activities. Her partner would frequently ask her to go to the movies, while RJ was unable to tolerate the feel of the seat cushions on her skin, the smell of the popcorn, and the loudness of the sound track. RJ could only eat at two restaurants in the neighboring area but preferred to eat at home. RJ could not understand her partner's frustration with her or her partner's need for physical affectionate contact. RJ was able to tolerate some sexual contact but avoided it whenever possible, as it was adverse to her but she understood from reading that it was an expected part of a relationship. After several months, RJ's partner terminated the relationship, much to RJ's relief. She was very happy to return home to her parents' house where she could have conversation with them at her initiative, and the expectations for social interaction or disruption of her schedule were minimal. It was comforting to return to her family's schedule, which she knew well. She did have the insight to know that her parents wouldn't always be there and knew that she needed to work earnestly to maintain at least some relationship with friends. She understood that even though it may be difficult to do so, she would have to initiate contact and not rely on her friends solely to initiate such contact.

The only significant predictor of romantic functioning among those with ASD is level of social functioning [21]. When meeting someone with ASD, several irregularities are noticeable. Persons with ASD frequently will not look into the eyes of the person with whom they are interacting; instead they may look at their mouths or perhaps even another object in the room [20]. Some of those with ASD would state that looking directly at another's person's eyes is extremely anxiety provoking, whereas others with ASD may be disinterested. Personal physical spatial boundaries, which many people take as second nature, are not part of the social make-up in persons with ASD. They may stand too close to a person with whom they may be interacting, or they may seem distant and uninvolved. Those with ASD may not pay attention to socially acceptable standards of personal appearance and may appear unkempt or inappropriately dressed for an occasion, e.g. wearing a casual, comfortable outfit to a formal event. Persons with ASD have a very difficult time engaging another person in conversation, i.e. they have difficulty initiating conversation or maintaining conversation through reciprocal social interaction [26]. A person with ASD may answer questions when asked or begin a scripted monologue that is repetitive in nature about an area of interest, with little to no awareness of the reaction of the person with whom they are interacting. Part of the reason for this lack of awareness is that a person with ASD is frequently unaware of the meaning of nonverbal behavior as a means of communication. The concept of theory of mind states that a person cannot understand the thoughts, intentions, and feelings of others or what another person means during an interaction, other than the concrete nature of the words stated [28]. For example, when a mother asked her child to "go sit in the tub", the child sat in the tub with all of her clothes on, when the mother of course meant to prepare for a bath. This may seem obvious to most people but might not be so obvious to a person with ASD. As a corollary, a person with ASD frequently cannot read the emotional meaning behind a verbal or nonverbal communication, i.e. interpret social cues [29]. A study by Izuma supports that people with autism lack the ability to take into consideration what others think of them [30]. Partially due to this lack of awareness, someone with ASD may respond in a very blunt or honest way to a statement of another person with whom they are interacting. For example, when asked a question such as "Do you like my new dress?", the person with ASD might say all the reasons they feel the dress is unattractive, being unaware of the emotional impact such statements might have on the person to whom they are making such comments [31].

6. Gender identity and sexual orientation

Gender identity usually develops in neurotypical children by the age of three [10] with ranges of 3-5 years of age [32]. Gender identity may be more rigid in individuals with ASD [33]. For children with developmental disabilities, gender identity in general likely develops in synchrony with many other developmental delays, especially in language, communication and social relatedness, which in turn influences the child's ability to mentally represent their own gender either in images or language. There is no current established literature about gender identity development in children with ASD; however, a recent article on gender dysphoria and identity difficulty found that clinics are reporting an overrepresentation of individuals with ASD in their gender identity referrals [33].

Sexual orientation refers to a person's established patterns of overall attraction to another person, including emotional, romantic, sexual, and behavioral attractions [34] regardless of whether this pattern results in sexual behavior. Research in the last several decades established sexual orientation on a continuum from entirely heterosexual, bisexual, and homosexual to asexual [35-37]. The relatively novel term "sexual fluidity" refers to the situation-dependent flexibility in someone's sexual responsiveness and may include both hetero- and same-sex experiences [37]. Same-sex behaviors among adolescents are reported between 5-10%, with similar percentages observed in adults [10].

Sexual identity develops normatively in adolescence related to puberty and overall body changes in the context of societal expectations about partner choices. For most adolescents with ASD, this development may occur later than that of their typically developing peers [38] and may include higher percentages of asexuality, but in most aspects of sexual development, the literature identifies similar desires and fantasies [21]. In fact, the literature on sexuality of children and adolescents with developmental disabilities cautions to not erroneously regard people with disabilities as childlike, asexual or as inappropriately sexual [39].

At the same time, several studies were identified by Healy and colleagues [19] that show that people with a disability may hold rather conservative views about their own sexuality related to negative caregiver attitudes toward certain sexual behaviors, including pre-marital sex and homosexual activity. Still, in comparison to caregiving staff, family members may altogether be less inclined to openly discuss issues of sexuality. Family members seemed to prefer low levels of intimacy in the relationships of their child amidst a high acceptance of platonic and non-intimate relationships [40].

7. ASD and intimacy

Individuals growing up with ASD have the same human needs for intimacy and relationships as anyone [41]. However, the self-identification of these needs may develop later than same age neurotypically developing peers and become expressed differently depending upon the individual's sexual knowledge, beliefs and values. Understanding of implicit dating rules and the hierarchy of sexual intimacies may become potential barriers for individuals with disabilities in general and particularly for adolescents and adults with ASD. Focus groups have been shown to make a difference in an individual's understanding, especially with involvement of his or her family and caregivers [19].

Intimacy is the sharing of emotional, cognitive and physical aspects of oneself with those of another. Individuals with ASD often have problems with rigidity and the need for repetition, which may limit the spontaneity and playfulness of sexual contact. Sensitivity to physical contact and inability to tolerate internal sensations created by physical intimacy may also create significant anxiety. The inability to read the thoughts, feelings, or expressed sensations of one's partner can lead to miscommunication, emotionally or physically painful experiences, and/or shame and guilt. In the context of navigating intimacy, by adulthood there are several options for types of relationships, typically to include living single, cohabitating with one or several others, and living in a marriage/partnership. Currently, many adult individuals with ASD continue to reside with their family of origin. Due to poor social relationships and lack of employment, living with family provides a comfortable social situation, as observed in the case of RJ. There is no need for continual social contact or concern for others, as family already exists as a group.

When even possible, marital relationships can be very strained, as the ASD spouse (usually a male) frequently has difficulty interpreting the spouse's need for emotional attention. Little to no research has been done on the adult lifestyles of higher functioning persons with ASD other than to say that most of them remain in their parents' home. Most previous research has been with those living in a residential setting. One study whose focus was to survey the gender identity of ASD subjects did ask a question pertaining to marital status. Gilmour and colleagues found that the group, which was atypically more female, did not differ from the control group on the basis of marital status. This result was unexpected and may be specific to the group surveyed of 82 persons with ASD [42]. More research is clearly needed in this area, but attaining accurate statistical data will be difficult, as many high functioning individuals with ASD are undiagnosed or misdiagnosed.

Case example: L

Patient, L is a 35-year-old male engineering student, who was accompanied by his wife for an initial assessment. L's wife believed that he had Asperger's disorder. He did not understand why this potential diagnosis would even matter to his wife. A major concern in their marriage was L's dislike for social situations. His wife worked at a bookstore and was frequently invited to her coworkers' houses to play games, watch movies, or perhaps have dinner. L would begrudgingly attend but would then sit quietly and not interact with anyone. His wife's friends would attempt to include him in conversations, but L would frequently give one-word answers and not reciprocate or would engage in a long monologue about his most recent engineering project. He did not understand his wife's distress at these situations. As a couple, it was their usual routine to have a date on Saturday night consisting of time spent together in an activity, followed by a sexual encounter. L did not understand why his wife would break this routine when she was upset by his lack of social interaction at her co-worker's home. He would become very angry and frustrated, slamming the door, and breaking small nearby items. His wife encouraged him to come to the appointment as a way for her to begin to understand his behavior and to find ways to cope with him.

8. Potential for abuse

For all individuals with disabilities, including ASD, there is an increased risk for physical and sexual abuse. In 2006, Murphy and Elias reported a sexual abuse rate that was 2.2 times higher than that of children without disabilities [39]. In a recent study, caregivers of individuals with autism reported that 16.6% had been sexually abused. Individuals with ASD can be subject to sexual victimization due to their trusting natures, desire to be socially accepted, lack of understanding of the meaning or possible consequences of their behavior, or exposure through internet contacts. Children who experienced sexual abuse were more likely to act out sexually or be sexually abusive toward others [43]. This mindset, although with seemingly honest intentions, places the ASD individual(s) at risk for sexual abuse, due to the lack of available sexual knowledge. Lack of knowledge can contribute to an individual not understanding appropriate boundaries and therefore they may not be able to distinguish when someone is touching them inappropriately. This, coupled with existing social deficits, has resulted in underreported sexual abuse in this population. Therefore, sexual education and public intervention strategies (which will be discussed later in this chapter) are key protective factors and could contribute to healthy sexual development.

Case example: M

A 17-year-old female patient, M, presented for diagnostic evaluation and was diagnosed with ASD. Her cognitive ability was in the low average IQ range. As a student in high school, she was very invested in making friends. She had difficulty managing the intricacies of relationships with other girls in her class, as her hygiene was below average and her clothing choices were not fashionable. M didn't belong to a specific social group of girls, such as cheerleaders, athletes, "Goths," etc. and therefore frequently sat by herself in the lunchroom. As she was failing in her social relationships with girls, she thought she would attempt to make friends with some of the boys in her class. She was coached by her younger sister at home (age 15 without ASD). Her sister was actually aware of M's poor social standing with other girls, as she was frequently asked what was wrong with her older sister by peers. M had previously made positive contact with a boy in her art class, who was drawing a video game character. The art teacher supported this interaction and facilitated their conversations in class. Her contact with another boy, however, was less than positive. He told M that the best way to make friends was to spend time together after school at the park. The boy then made sexual advances, kissing the patient. She was very confused and did not stop his behavior, which led him to attempt to fondle her genital area. The encounter stopped at that point. M did not bring this event to the attention of her parents or sister. Fortunately, in her therapy session, she was able to ask if it was OK for a boy to put his hand in her pants. Clearly, M had not received instruction from her parents about "appropriate touch." The parents brought this situation to the attention of the school administrators, who reprimanded the boy but could not address it further, as M was older than 16 and it was deemed that she consented to the behavior by not stopping him.

9. Inappropriate sexual behavior

Along with the concerns of interpersonal intimacy and delayed maturity of sexuality, individuals with ASD may have difficulty determining what and where sexual behaviors are appropriate. Permitted behavior is governed by social appropriateness, which is gathered through social cues. With the limited ability to read and understand social cues, those with an ASD diagnosis can fail to discern between acceptable public behavior and acceptable private behavior [44]. A review article by Stokes and Kaur included masturbatory behaviors in public, removing clothing in public, and touching members of the opposite sex, as reported in previous studies, followed sometimes by the rejection of others due to these problematic behaviors [45]. For example, masturbatory activities are often seen in public when anxiety levels have increased. This in turn could potentially lead to legal implications. Among adolescents with ASD, some concerns include inappropriate courting behaviors, such as stalking or touching the person of interest inappropriately, making inappropriate comments, not always understanding the need for privacy such as knocking on doors [45], making threats against the person of interest, or exhibiting obsessive interest in a person [21], which can lead to both interpersonal and legal consequences. Behavioral and educational interventions must be considered in order to serve as a protective buffer against undesired outcomes.

Case example: C

Patient C is a 14-year-old boy diagnosed with autism who had minimal verbal skills. At age 14, he was 6'2" tall. Cognitively, he was functioning at the mild intellectual disability range (IQ ~70). C had no friends. His social judgment was poor, so his parents encouraged his interactions and visits with extended family in an effort to improve his social communication. One of the patient's areas of interest was wrestling. He would frequently roughhouse with his other male cousins, who were teenagers as well. On one visit, C was watching a wrestling program with his younger cousin, age 4, as the older boys had gone to the movies and C refused to attend. C, not understanding the social implications of his behavior, began to roughhouse with his young cousin. When his mother and aunt entered the room, C was laying on top of his 4-year-old cousin in what was judged to be an attempt by the patient to molest this young child, whereas C thought he had won the wrestling match like the man on television. When asked, C could not adequately explain his behavior, due to his limited verbal skills. His mother was able to reassure the young boy's mother that C had no sexual intent. However, C and his mother no longer received invitations to visit the home of those relatives.

Masturbation especially in public settings has been the central focus within the developmental disorder literature due to the concerns and personal views of the general public and legal officials. In particular, these groups possess a tendency to label public masturbation as sexual deviancy. This predisposition was greatly reduced when both groups received training on the behaviors of individuals with ASD.

10. Sexual education

Sexual education is a core ingredient of successful intervention beginning with body anatomy, physiology and personal hygiene, taught in childhood. As the individual with ASD reaches older adolescence and adulthood, social dictates of what is appropriate sexual behavior in public must be carefully taught with video modeling and social stories [23] to prevent problematic outcomes for the person with ASD and those around him or her [21]. As with all stages of development, sexual development may be delayed, while pubertal development may be chronologically on time. The family needs to be educated about teaching sexuality as well in order to facilitate the knowledge of the individual with ASD throughout his or her development [8,44]. Sexual education can also prevent sexual abuse, unwanted pregnancies, and sexually transmitted infections, or STI [8]. A recent article on the sexuality of children and adolescents identified educational needs in the context of parent and health care professionals' expectations [39]. Likewise, a greater educational need was identified for caregivers of individuals with disabilities to help individual better navigate their social environment with implemented help on a societal and political level [44,46,47]. DeLamater and Friedrich cited the Kaiser Family Foundation (1997), noting that young people especially name mass media as a primary source of information about sex and intimacy over information and education provided by parents or professionals [10].

This is likely even more true currently, with youth having increased access to information via the Internet and the use of personal electronics. In this sense, the use of electronics may become a useful educational medium and perhaps even an interactive tool to facilitate development of socially expected courting and dating behaviors, with the goal of becoming able to establish longer term romantic relationships.

Education about sexuality is critical for the ASD population. Many persons with ASD have the desire to have friendships and intimate relationships; however it is very difficult for them to make the complex emotional distinctions between friendship, kindness, and romantic interest. In a study by Hellemans, the majority of subjects with ASD expressed sexual interest but lacked the appropriate skills and knowledge to have a successful relationship [48]. Their misinterpretations can lead to emotional pain for themselves and possibly inappropriate behaviors toward others [26]. The most common forms of sexuality education for adolescents and young adults occur through conversations with their peers and/or their families. A study by Realmuto and Ruble suggested that typical children learn about sexuality via casual social experiences, including those in the community, family and school settings [49]. Persons with ASD are at a unique disadvantage as they do not initiate or maintain social contacts to acquire such education. Family members approach sexuality in their children with ASD by denying it and not teaching sexuality at all, or by considering that their ASD children can approach sexuality as any other adolescent would [21]. In a study by Stokes and colleagues, 25 subjects with ASD aged 13-36 were compared to a normal control group of the same age; the study found that persons with ASD relied less upon peers and friends for knowledge but relied more on information they learned through reading and other similar activities [21].

When considering education about sexuality, three content areas need to be included: 1) basic facts and accurate information, 2) formation of individual values with consideration of family values, and 3) application of sexuality to relationships and social situations [15]. More specifically, basic biology of the sexual organs and how they function for males and females, maintenance of hygiene, prevention of pregnancy and sexually transmitted diseases, methods of birth control, how to initiate and maintain intimate sexual relationships, how to prevent unwanted sexual contact, the role of masturbation as a normal sexual bodily function and its social implications, as well as reproductive and parenting rights. What is most essential is to maintain a consistent focus on the social component of sexual behavior [8]. Due to theory of mind deficits, a person with ASD may be unable to understand the actions, feelings and intentions of others, such as not recognizing obvious clues of disinterest and being inappropriately persistent in pursuing a desired person. The person with ASD must learn how to initiate romantic relationships, understand dating behaviors, know appropriate physical boundaries, develop listening skills, and understand the meaning of consensual sexual activity [8]. Frequently, booster sessions are recommended as an individual grows and develops and has the need for additional information and skills or reinforcement of principles already learned that may have been forgotten [8].

Deciding who should teach a person with ASD about sexuality can be confusing. A team approach may be most successful. Parents and caregivers usually provide primary instruction but may need the support of a formal sexual education program provided by the school system. Parents provide the foundation for the development of the child's sexuality by modeling relationships in the home. The family's moral values, culture, religion, and other beliefs are clearly a major part of sexuality education. An IEP team can designate a specific component of the health curriculum to sexuality that must be geared to the child's cognitive, emotional, and social level of development. Such a plan should be revisited and revised as a child/adolescent matures with the need for more information, skills, and attitudes [8].

11. Model programs

Several models and approaches to sexuality education for those with ASD have been published. One model from a research study in Israel provided treatment through ten bi-weekly sessions, each devoted to topics that included establishment of self-identity, acceptance of one's disability, independence in social life, establishment of friendship and intimate relationships, sexual knowledge and development, and safety skills [50]. The aims of the group were to 1) discuss attitudes and feelings, 2) provide information, 3) advise parents on how to help children manage their sexuality, and 4) encourage independence in their children. The overarching principles of this group treatment were to 1) develop an appropriate self-concept, 2) find a similar social group, 3) develop relations based on equality and reciprocity, and 4) prevent abusive relations, with all of these aims potentially leading to satisfactory intimate romantic relationships. The most improvement in this study was shown in social development and the development of a clearer concept of friendship.

Case example: H

H is a 19-year-old female who recently began attending community college. She has an above average IQ and good facility with language. She was able to manage some friendships in high school by being the manager of one of the girls' sports teams. The girls on the team were kind to her and included her in team activities, encouraged by the team's coach. H also belonged to the Anime club and had some friends there. The structured schedule of high school, along with the academic supports provided by her Individualized education plan, coaching and encouragement from her parents, enabled her success. H was having a difficult transition to college with no friends, no academic supports, and a less structured schedule. She attended a session provided by the disability services department and sat next to a boy several years older than she with a similar disability, who initiated and maintained a conversation. H was aware that he was a stranger and was careful in the information she provided. He asked her to meet for lunch at the cafeteria several times. H's mother wanted to meet him because she was unsure of her daughter's social judgment. With her parent's approval and her mother's coaching about dating, they went to a movie. Their relationship slowly progressed over the last six months beyond the handholding stage to the first kiss. H's boyfriend was able to allow her to manage the relationship to assist H in dealing with the anxiety that this relationship had created for her, though she was beginning to increasingly enjoy their time together.

Another intervention that shows promise is the development of Social Stories™ by Carol Gray [51] which can be tailored to each child or adult and written in the person's perspective, so it can be used to prepare persons for dealing with friendships, managing intimacy, and improving safety [23]. Video modeling is another technique where a student watches a video where peers or others demonstrate appropriate behavior. The student then models the behavior he or she just viewed. Video modeling, by providing some distance, helps relieve some anxiety during a practice phase before trying a real time interaction [23].

Concepts from other treatment centers have added to sexuality education. Two precepts from the Devereaux Centers for Autism emphasize that 1) parents are the best sexual educators and 2) it is normal and natural for every person with a body to express their sexuality regardless of their disability [44]. The Benhaven residential program for those with autism emphasizes 1) the need to teach students socially acceptable sexual behavior appropriate for both childhood and adulthood 2) no disapproval of masturbation when done in socially appropriate situations as it may be the only sexual satisfaction some individuals with autism may experience and 3) do not encourage behavior beyond which an individual is capable or that will lead to frustration and disappointment [44].

It is helpful to consider the basic learning needs of those with ASD in general and apply them to sexuality education [26].

1. Use of visual aids, role play

2. Use of concrete, specific examples instead of abstract concepts

3. Dividing large blocks of information into smaller, sequential segments

4. Allowing time for comments and questions

5. Keeping brief any discussions of feelings so as not to confuse or overwhelm

6. Provide overviews and structure to the lesson

7. Include specific problem solving strategies and examples

Especially when considering sexuality education in those with lower functioning ASD, the capacity to make sexually-related decisions must be considered. A study of four adults with moderate intellectual disability (not autism) focused on improving capacity to make sexuality related decisions [52]. Treatment was rendered on a 1:1 basis for 20 sessions. The article by Dukes and colleagues emphasizes that in order to provide valid consent to sexual contact, the person with a disability requires knowledge about sexuality and the understanding of the concept of what is and is not voluntary [52]. Consent must also be individualized and situation specific for decision-making associated with sexual contact. This intervention focused on sexual safety practices, knowledge of the physical self, knowledge of sexual functioning, and knowledge of choices and consequences in sexual matters. The study noted the need for booster sessions, as the memory of topics covered waned with time, perhaps secondary to little opportunity to utilize the information learned [52]. A survey of the sexual behavior of 89 adults with autism living in group homes in North Carolina found that the majority of individuals were engaging in some form of sexual behavior [53], with masturbation being the most common sexual behavior. One third of the residents did have other oriented sexual behavior, which mostly consisted of holding hands, touching, and kissing. One third of the residents did not masturbate at all. A major concern with lower functioning individuals is the inappropriate expression of sexual behaviors in a socially unacceptable manner [53].

To improve decision-making related to sexuality in individuals with an intellectual disability, Dukes and McGuire adapted successfully a sexual education program for individuals with special needs called Living Your Life [52]. Possibly such a program could also further be adapted to the specific knowledge and needs of individuals with ASD. In their 2010 article, Travers and Tincani identified Body Awareness, Social Development, Romantic Relationships and Intimacy, Masturbation and Modifying Behavior to Meet Social Norms, and Reproductive and Parenting Rights of Individuals with ASD as crucial components of sexuality education for individuals with ASD [8]. These authors also identified the need for professionals to address sexuality education in an open, confident, and objective manner in a collaborative effort with the individual with ASD and their family.

The TEACCH program [54] has explicit guidelines for teaching sexuality education to the lower functioning person with ASD [16]. An important component is taking an individualized developmental approach, with the goal of matching teaching programs to level of function and development of long range goals (e.g. capacity to have a romantic relationship versus ability to enjoy masturbation in a socially acceptable manner). Another concept is that sexuality cannot be taught in isolation but must be considered in the context of other skills, such as one's ability to verbally communicate or one's cognitive ability, The most basic skill is the ability to have discriminate learning, for example, knowing where and when to touch others or masturbate, and can be taught from a behavioral perspective, with rewards for appropriate behavior. Environmental supports to reinforce appropriate behaviors can be very useful, and environmental changes (e.g. wearing a belt to help prevent a young man from masturbating in public) may allow for intervention prior to a behavior occurring, as slowing down the behavior provides more time to intervene. The next level beyond discriminate learning is managing personal hygiene, followed by understanding body parts and their functions. The highest level is a complete sex education program, including development of sexual relationships with others.

Social skills groups and meet-ups for older adolescents and young adults are essential to continue to build on social skills and allow for facilitated interaction [55]. A recent study with adolescents and young adults with ASD by Stokes and colleagues found that one's level of social functioning predicted romantic functioning [21]. The development of social interaction skills will help promote interest in developing meaningful relationships with others that in turn may lead to intimate relationships and ultimately more independent living arrangements. Equally important are the development of emotion regulation and self-esteem skills that will help to navigate difficulties and changes within significant relationships. In their 2006 article, Murphy and Elias [39] described how children and adolescents with disabilities generally have fewer skills and opportunities to engage in social interactions that could lead potentially into intimate relationships. In particular, this important article emphasizes particular skills that are often amiss for individuals with disabilities, Abilities, especially the ability to make eye contact, develop appropriate greetings, recognize personal space, and interpret nonverbal communication, that apply to individuals with ASD [39].

Based on previous studies, and addressing the gap in identified interventions specific to the sexual development of individuals with ASD, a current intervention program called Growing Up Aware is in the process of being developed at Columbia University [14]. The first research component attempted to better understand how parents teach their children with ASD about sexuality. Results of the study showed that the majority of parents indicated a strong interest in learning how to better communicate with their children about sexual and reproductive health [14]. This is met currently by insufficient availability of materials for parents. Many clinical providers appear under-equipped, with normative knowledge and skills themselves about how to address questions of parents regarding their child's changing sexual development based on parental perception. Clinicians need to become better equipped to help families with unusual or inappropriate sexual development.

12. Medication concerns

Medication side effects that were not troubling to a child with ASD may cause significant distress in an adult with ASD by decreasing sexual desire or interfering with sexual potency [56]. Self-injury may result if appropriate instruction about masturbation is not provided. Medications such as fluoxetine or sertraline (selective serotonin reuptake inhibitors) are frequently prescribed for persons with ASD to help with anxiety or repetitive behaviors. This group of medications can cause a decrease in sexual desire or make it much more difficult to attain an orgasm. Since masturbation is one of the most frequent sexual behaviors within the ASD population, unintentional self-injury may result from prolonged attempts to reach orgasm. Appropriate instruction in masturbatory behaviors may be necessary in order to prevent self-injury [46]. Alternately, a medication with sexual side effects may be beneficial for a patient who has anxiety and/or excessive inappropriate sexual behaviors by decreasing sexual desire [57] and enhancing the effectiveness of behavioral interventions.

13. Public intervention

There are many important reasons for promoting sexuality education for those with ASD including the following: 1) prevention of sexual abuse, 2) preventing inappropriate sexual behavior toward others, 3) promoting health and hygiene and preventing sexually transmitted disease and pregnancy, 4) facilitating the development of intimate relationships, and 5) preventing self-injury [8]. A basic tenet is that sexuality education for persons with ASD must be geared to their particular level of cognitive, emotional, and social functioning and is most effective when it is highly individualized. Those with ASD have a right to have a sexual life, a right to receive guidance and support, and they need assistance in expressing sexuality in an acceptable way to those in their environment [8].

Public intervention strategies should primarily focus on educating the community about the behaviors and traits common to persons with Autism Spectrum Disorders. Education has been shown to foster tolerance and understanding. In addition to this, education tends to spawn advocacy, thereby facilitating the needed changes in existing policies and law. In particular, advocates of those with ASD have the greatest opportunity to teach others about this population by modeling how best to support persons with ASD in the community.

Particular attention should be given to law enforcement, judicial systems and other populations that traditionally have minimal contact with individuals with ASD [7]. Educational efforts should include a discussion of basic symptomatology, behavioral interventions and treatments. Efforts should also be made to dispel myths, misconceptions and assumptions about those with ASD [58]. In addition, education should include information about potential risks to this population and the available programs and systems that are in place to provide protection for the ASD population [44].

14. Conclusion

In summary, our literature review and ample experiences of the families in our clinical practice show that, while every person has the innate basis for developing sexuality in a multitude of expressions and experiences, individuals with disabilities (and especially individuals with an Autism Spectrum Disorder) most often require additional education and help to become able to express their sexuality in a socially appropriate way. While most neurotypically developing peers form intimate relationships beginning in adolescence and into adulthood, along a variety of experiences from dating to partnering in committed relationships, many individuals with an Autism Spectrum Disorder remain living with their family of origin into their adulthood and have significant difficulty navigating the social expectations surrounding relationships. Their difficulty may pertain to recognizing their own needs and wants, as well as to recognizing their partner's wishes coupled with more inexperience than their peers in this arena. Individuals with ASD and their parents and caregivers frequently identify this difficulty when directly asked about it. Sexuality education in a supportive format that includes the individual's family and their particular values and background will be most effective. Interventions need to be individualized with a long-range goal that matches the cognitive, social, and emotional developmental level of the person with ASD. As the prevalence of persons with ASD increases in our society, we are more than ever called to support their ability to mature into adults capable of functioning in all areas of life, including sexuality and intimacy.

Author details

Maria R. Urbano, Kathrin Hartmann, Stephen I. Deutsch, Gina M. Bondi Polychronopoulos and Vanessa Dorbin

*Address all correspondence to: urbanomr@evms.edu

Department of Psychiatry and Behavioral Sciences, Eastern Virginia Medical School, Norfolk, Virginia, USA

References

[1] Association AP. Diagnostic and Statistical Manual of Mental Disorders (fourth ed., text rev.). Washington, DC: Author; 2000.

[2] American Psychological Association http://www.apa.org2012.

[3] Frazier TW, Youngstrom EA, Speer L, Embacher R, Law P, Constantino J, et al. Validation of proposed DSM-5 criteria for autism spectrum disorder. J Am Acad Child Adolesc Psychiatry. 2012 Jan;51(1):28-40.e3. PubMed PMID: 22176937. Pubmed Central PMCID: PMC3244681. eng.

[4] Mandy WP, Charman T, Skuse DH. Testing the construct validity of proposed criteria for DSM-5 autism spectrum disorder. J Am Acad Child Adolesc Psychiatry. 2012 Jan;51(1):41-50. PubMed PMID: 22176938. eng.

[5] Prevalence of Autism Spectrum Disorders-Autism and Developmental Disabilities Monitoring Network, 14 sites, US 2008. Surveillance Summaries March 30, 2012. Morbidity and Mortality Weekly Report 61(SS03) 1-19.

[6] CDC. Morbidity and Mortality Weekly Report 2012; 61(SS--3): [1-19 pp.].

[7] McCarthy M. Women with Intellectual Disabilities: Finding a Place in the World. Traustadottir RJ, K., editor. London, England: Jessica Kingsley Publishers; 2000.

[8] Travers J, Tincani M. Sexuality education for individuals with Autism Spectrum Disorders: Critical issues and decision making guidelines. Education and Training in Autism and Developmental Disabilities. 2010;45(2):284-93.

[9] Freud A. The Concept of Developmental Lines. Psychoanal Study Child. 1963;18:245-65. PubMed PMID: 14147280. eng.

[10] DeLamater J, Friedrich WN. Human sexual development. J Sex Res. 2002 Feb;39(1): 10-4. PubMed PMID: 12476250. eng.

[11] CDC. Trends in the prevalence of sexual behavior and HIV testing: National YRBS 1991-2011. http://www.cdc.gov/healthyyouth/yrbs/pdf/us_sexual_trend_yrbs.pdf: 2011.

[12] Nussey SS, Whitehead, SA. Endocrinology: An Integrated Approach. Oxford: Bios Scientific Publishers; 2001.

[13] Erikson E. Childhood and Society. New York: Norton; 1950.

[14] Ballan MS. Parental perspectives of communication about sexuality in families of children with autism spectrum disorders. J Autism Dev Disord. 2012 May;42(5): 676-84. PubMed PMID: 21681591. eng.

[15] Gerhardt, P. Sexuality Instruciton and Autism Spectrum Disorders: Autism Society. Copyright 2006-2012. Education.com. All rights reserved. http://www.education.com/reference/article/sexuality-instruction-autism-ASD/

[16] Sexuality and Autism. TEACCH Report. Autism independent UK. http:www.autismuk.com/index9sub1.htm

[17] Mesibov G, Schopler E. Autism in Adolescents and Adults. New York: Plenum Press; 1983.

[18] Klinger L, Dawson G, Renner P. Autistic Disorder. In: Mash E, Barkley R, editors. Child Psychopathology. 2nd ed. New York: Guilford Press; 2003.

[19] Healy E, McGuire BE, Evans DS, Carley SN. Sexuality and personal relationships for people with an intellectual disability. Part I: service-user perspectives. J Intellect Disabil Res. 2009 Nov;53(11):905-12. PubMed PMID: 19709348. eng.

[20] McPartland JC, Pelphrey KA. The Implications of Social Neuroscience for Social Disability. J Autism Dev Disord. 2012 Mar. PubMed PMID: 22456816. ENG.

[21] Stokes M, Newton N, Kaur A. Stalking, and social and romantic functioning among adolescents and adults with autism spectrum disorder. J Autism Dev Disord. 2007 Nov;37(10):1969-86. PubMed PMID: 17273936. eng.

[22] Shandra CL, Chowdhury AR. The first sexual experience among adolescent girls with and without disabilities. J Youth Adolesc. 2012 Apr;41(4):515-32. PubMed PMID: 21559882. eng.

[23] Chan J, John RM. Sexuality and sexual health in children and adolescents with autism. The Journal for Nurse Practitioners. 2012;8(4):306-15.

[24] Perry N. Adults on the Autism Spectrum leave the nest: Achieving Supported Independence: Jessica Kingsley Publishers; 2009.

[25] Losh M, Capps L. Understanding of emotional experience in autism: insights from the personal accounts of high-functioning children with autism. Dev Psychol. 2006 Sep;42(5):809-18. PubMed PMID: 16953688. eng.

[26] Ray F, Marks C, Bray-Garretson H. Challenges to treating adolescents with Asperger's Syndrome who are sexually abusive. Sexual Addiction & Compulsivity. 2004;11:264-85.

[27] Stichter JP, Herzog MJ, Visovsky K, Schmidt C, Randolph J, Schultz T, et al. Social competence intervention for youth with Asperger Syndrome and high-functioning autism: an initial investigation. J Autism Dev Disord. 2010 Sep;40(9):1067-79. PubMed PMID: 20162344. eng.

[28] Baron-Cohen S, Leslie AM, Frith U. Does the autistic child have a "theory of mind"? Cognition. 1985 Oct;21(1):37-46. PubMed PMID: 2934210. eng.

[29] Jellema T, Lorteije J, van Rijn S, van t' Wout M, de Haan E, van Engeland H, et al. Involuntary interpretation of social cues is compromised in autism spectrum disorders. Autism Res. 2009 Aug;2(4):192-204. PubMed PMID: 19642087. eng.

[30] Izuma K, Matsumoto K, Camerer CF, Adolphs R. Insensitivity to social reputation in autism. Proc Natl Acad Sci U S A. 2011 Oct;108(42):17302-7. PubMed PMID: 21987799. Pubmed Central PMCID: PMC3198313. eng.

[31] Bauminger N. The facilitation of social-emotional understanding and social interaction in high-functioning children with autism: intervention outcomes. J Autism Dev Disord. 2002 Aug;32(4):283-98. PubMed PMID: 12199133. eng.

[32] Ruble DN, Taylor LJ, Cyphers L, Greulich FK, Lurye LE, Shrout PE. The role of gender constancy in early gender development. Child Dev. 2007 2007 Jul-Aug; 78(4):1121-36. PubMed PMID: 17650129. eng.

[33] de Vries AL, Noens IL, Cohen-Kettenis PT, van Berckelaer-Onnes IA, Doreleijers TA. Autism spectrum disorders in gender dysphoric children and adolescents. J Autism Dev Disord. 2010 Aug;40(8):930-6. PubMed PMID: 20094764. Pubmed Central PMCID: PMC2904453. eng.

[34] Division 44/Committee on Lesbian G, and Bisexual Concerns Joint Task Force on Guidelines for Psychotherapy with Lesbian, G.y, and Bisexual Clients. Guidelines for psychotherapy with lesbian, gay, and bisexual clients. Am Psychol. 2000 Dec; 55(12):1440-51. PubMed PMID: 11260872. eng.

[35] Kinsey AC, Pomeroy WB, Martin CE. Sexual behavior in the human male. Philadelphia: W.B. Saunders; 1948.

[36] Klein F. The bisexual option. New York: Harrington Park Press; 1993.

[37] Diamond LM. Sexual fluidity: Understanding women's love and desire. Cambridge, Mass.: Harvard University Press; 2008.

[38] Volkmar FR, Carter A, Sparrow SS, Cicchetti DV. Quantifying social development in autism. J Am Acad Child Adolesc Psychiatry. 1993 May;32(3):627-32. PubMed PMID: 7684364. eng.

[39] Murphy NA, Elias ER. Sexuality of children and adolescents with developmental disabilities. Pediatrics. 2006 Jul;118(1):398-403. PubMed PMID: 16818589. eng.

[40] Evans DE, Rothbart MK. A Two-Factor Model of Temperament. Pers Individ Dif. 2009 Oct;47(6):565-70. PubMed PMID: 20161172. Pubmed Central PMCID: PMC2722842. ENG.

[41] Ousley OY, Mesibov GB. Sexual attitudes and knowledge of high-functioning adolescents and adults with autism. J Autism Dev Disord. 1991 Dec;21(4):471-81. PubMed PMID: 1778961. eng.

[42] Gilmour L, Schalomon PM, Smith V. Sexuality in a community based sample of adults with Autism Spectrum Disorder. Research in Autism Spectrum Disorders. 2012;6:313-8.

[43] Mandell DS, Walrath CM, Manteuffel B, Sgro G, Pinto-Martin JA. The prevalence and correlates of abuse among children with autism served in comprehensive community-based mental health settings. Child Abuse Negl. 2005 Dec;29(12):1359-72. PubMed PMID: 16293306. eng.

[44] Koller R. Sexuality and Adolescents with Autism. Sexuality and Disability. 2000;18(2):125-35.

[45] Stokes M, Kaur A. High Functioning Autism and Sexuality: A Parental Perspective. Autism. 2005;9(3):266-89.

[46] McGuire BE, Bayley AA. Relationships, sexuality and decision-making capacity in people with an intellectual disability. Current Opinion in Psychiatry. 2011;24:398-402.

[47] Kandel I, Morad M, Vardi G, Merrick J. Intellectual disability and parenthood. Scientific World Journal. 2005 Jan;5:50-7. PubMed PMID: 15674450. eng.

[48] Hellemans H, Colson K, Verbraeken C, Vermeiren R, Deboutte D. Sexual behavior in high-functioning male adolescents and young adults with autism spectrum disorder. J Autism Dev Disord. 2007 Feb;37(2):260-9. PubMed PMID: 16868848. eng.

[49] Realmuto GM, Ruble LA. Sexual behaviors in autism: problems of definition and management. J Autism Dev Disord. 1999 Apr;29(2):121-7. PubMed PMID: 10382132. eng.

[50] Plaks M, Argaman R, Stawski M, Qwiat T, Polak D, Gothelf D. Social-sexual education in adolescents with behavioral neurogenetic syndromes. Isr J Psychiatry Relat Sci. 2010;47(2):118-24. PubMed PMID: 20733254. eng.

[51] Gray C. The New Social Story Book. Arlington, Texas: Future Horizons, Inc.; 2010.

[52] Dukes E, McGuire BE. Enhancing capacity to make sexuality-related decisions in people with an intellectual disability. J Intellect Disabil Res. 2009 Aug;53(8):727-34. PubMed PMID: 19527433. eng.

[53] Van Bourgondien ME, Reichle NC, Palmer A. Sexual behavior in adults with autism. J Autism Dev Disord. 1997 Apr;27(2):113-25. PubMed PMID: 9105963. eng.

[54] Haracopos D, Pederson L. Danish Report. Sexuality and Autism [Internet]. 1992.

[55] White SW, Albano AM, Johnson CR, Kasari C, Ollendick T, Klin A, et al. Development of a cognitive-behavioral intervention program to treat anxiety and social deficits in teens with high-functioning autism. Clin Child Fam Psychol Rev. 2010 Mar; 13(1):77-90. PubMed PMID: 20091348. Pubmed Central PMCID: PMC2863047. eng.

[56] Physicians Desk Reference. 66 ed. Montvale, NJ: Thomson PDR; 2012.

[57] Albertini G, Polito E, Sarà M, Di Gennaro G, Onorati P. Compulsive masturbation in infantile autism treated by mirtazapine. Pediatr Neurol. 2006 May;34(5):417-8. PubMed PMID: 16648008. eng.

[58] Irvine A. Issues in sexuality for individuals with developmental disabilities: Myths, misconceptions, and mistreatment. Exceptionality Education Canada. 2005;15(3): 5-20.

Chapter 4

Autism Spectrum Disorders in People with Sensory and Intellectual Disabilities Symptom Overlap and Differentiating Characteristics

Gitta De Vaan, Mathijs P.J. Vervloed,
Harry Knoors and Ludo Verhoeven

Additional information is available at the end of the chapter

1. Introduction

Autism Spectrum Disorders (ASD) are developmental disorders that people are burdened with for their whole life. They origin in childhood and are featured by restrictions in social and emotional development, communication, interests and motor skills [1]. People with autism are characterized by three major deficits as defined by the most recent version of diagnostic and statistical manual of mental disorders (DSM-IV-TR). These deficits include qualitative impairments in social interaction, qualitative impairments in communication and restricted, repetitive and stereotyped patterns of behaviour [2]. Behaviours within these main components of ASD may differ per individual because they are expressed in unique ways for each individual. Variations can be found in the way, the intensity and the perseverance with which the symptoms are expressed. Also the core characteristics may vary per individual. Where skills, interests and intellectual levels differ between people, so do the characteristics of autism, only the main problem areas remain the same [3]. In the current chapter, not only autism as defined by DSM-IV-TR, but also all variations within the autistic spectrum will be included.

Several symptoms of ASD are not unique but also found in other groups of people with disabilities. Similar behaviours, overlapping symptoms, or even the exact same behavioural characteristics can be found in people with hearing disabilities [4], visual impairments [5], intellectual disabilities [6] and combinations of these impairments, such as deafblindness [7]. All three of the main components of autism that the DSM-IV-TR describes, are also found in non autistic people with sensory and intellectual disabilities.

Furthermore, the prevalence of ASD seems to be much higher in people with one or more of these disabilities. In the entire population ASD is estimated to occur in at least between 0,1 and 0,6 percent [8, 9] and at most 2,64 percent [10]. In people with intellectual disabilities reported prevalences are much higher, ranging from 4 up to 60 percent [11]. Without giving exact rates the prevalence of ASD and autistic features in people with sensory disabilities is reported to be much higher than in typically developing people [12-14] It is an interesting question what cause this increase in prevalence when other impairments are involved. An obvious explanation could be a relationship between ASD and sensory or intellectual disabilities. An alternative explanation is an overlap of symptoms, but not of the underlying mechanisms, between autistic people without other disabilities and people with sensory and intellectual impairments. If the latter is the case, some people might be unfairly diagnosed as autistic when in fact they are not. False positive diagnoses then causes the increase in prevalence of ASD in sensory, intellectually and multiply impaired people.

The overlap in symptoms between people with ASD and people with sensory, intellectual and multiple impairments interferes with the right classification of the behaviour of people with sensory and intellectual disabilities. Several authors stress that even though the symptoms are similar, the processes that underlie these symptoms are different for autistic versus non autistic people [4, 15, 16]. Nevertheless, when behaviours are the same, there is the risk that ASD is either missed or unjustly diagnosed. A wrong classification may lead to a wrong treatment plan, which is especially problematic if the treatment plan is counterproductive for the true underlying cause. A treatment is most effective if it tackles the cause of the behaviours. An example is the stopping of stereotyped movements. Whereas in the blind these are usually caused by a lack of stimulation from the environment [17, 18], in people with ASD stereotyped movements can occur to get away from too much stimulation from the environment [19, 20].

The current chapter will give a comprehensive overview of the overlapping symptoms between autistic and non autistic people; it will elaborate on the categories that the DSM-IV-TR distinguishes as well as on the overlap within these categories for autistic and non-autistic people, it will describe the differences between the two groups and finally explain why a better differentiation is necessary.

2. Qualitative impairments in social interaction

The first characteristic of autism, according to DSM-IV-TR is defined as qualitative impairments in social interaction. These impairments can express through a variety of symptoms: problems in reciprocity and sharing of interests and emotions; impairments in non-verbal behaviours and impairments in joint attention, either in sharing, following or directing [2]. All of these problems in social behaviours contribute to problems in the development of proper peer relations.

2.1. Reciprocity and peer relationships

Some children with ASD prefer doing things alone and might avoid all kinds of social play [2]. Lack of reciprocity is also shown in an aversion to social touch and in problems with responding to your own name [21]. In young children impairments in this area are often expressed as inappropriate responses towards other people and being more interested in objects than people [19].

Autistic people may find it difficult to engage in peer relationships. However, they are not the only ones that have trouble in this area. A recent study about the popularity of deaf children showed that deaf children were less accepted and less popular than their hearing peers. This was explained by them being, amongst others variables, more withdrawn, less prosocial and worse at monitoring a conversation [22], behaviours also typical for ASD in a hearing population.

People with intellectual disabilities show problems in the area of reciprocity and relationships too. Often, intellectual disabilities are caused by abnormalities in the brain. It is not surprising to find that these abnormalities cause problems in people's emotional and social behaviours. However, not everyone with serious intellectual disabilities has social or emotional problems, some of them are even overly interested in social contact. Reciprocity and engagement are definitely present while communicating with them [3]. According to Wing [23] one can spot the difference between impaired social behaviour in intellectually impaired people with ASD versus intellectually impaired people without ASD by looking at the severity of the social impairments.

The problems in reciprocity and developing relationships are not limited to people with ASD, and auditory or mental disabilities. In 1977 Selma Fraiberg described the development of blind children. She noticed that blind children do not reach out to their parents as much as their sighted peers do. This may appear as a lack of reciprocity, when in fact seeing a parent makes sighted children reach out. Blind children obviously lack this ability [24]. This explains their less frequent attempts in reaching out, without any relationship with reciprocity. Moreover, according to Fraiberg, the absence of reaching out could make parents less responsive to their children, restraining them in their development of relationships. She explains that in the sighted, the smallest amount of eye contact with a baby can make an adult talk or play with them [24]. When signals such as reaching out and making eye contact are absent, the development of reciprocity and relationships could be impaired because of this. In fact, because the care for a blind child is so much more challenging and reciprocal signals are easily missed, lack of vision may increase the risk of problems in attachment [18]. However, Warren stressed that despite an increased risk, attachment problems can be avoided if the parents of a blind child respond appropriately. Assessing attachment highlights another problem, that is the reliability and validity of assessment instruments and procedures in children with disabilities. Attachment in sighted children is often tested by the strange situation method [25] where a child's reaction upon reunion with its mother is assessed after it has been left alone or in the presence of a stranger. Children with visual impairments, especially blind children, may not notice the departure and reappearance of their mother and may therefore fail to respond like sighted children would do [18]. In this case the perception problems interfere with possible affirmations of attachment problems. The same problems occur when observing people whilst looking for signals of reciprocity or interest in other people. Because of a loss of sight children with visual impairment or blindness may not notice other people or other people's behaviour. In extreme cases they do not show any interest in their surroundings because of poor vision and direct all their attention to objects within arm's reach or to their own body. This is especially the case in deafblind children who have not only problems in vision but also hearing, the two distant senses. Their remaining senses (touch, smell, taste and proprioception) only function in nearby space, giving the impression that deafblind children are ego-centred. This ego-centeredness is however of a different origin than it is in ASD [4].

2.2. Verbal and non-verbal social behaviours

In people with ASD, much verbal and non-verbal behaviour is impaired. This can express itself in to unnatural eye-to-eye gaze, a failure to correctly understand and execute facial expressions, atypical body postures and gestures to regulate social interaction. People with ASD often show less eye contact and fewer social smiles to others. They may also show problems in understanding facial expressions and the underlying emotions [19].

Non-verbal behaviours are very important in social communication and are used to make messages more clear. It's hard to imagine communicating without facial expressions, gestures, posture or understanding gaze direction. People with impairments miss a lot of these signals while communicating. In a visually impaired group it may be hard to distinguish autistic people from non-autistic people based on non-verbal behaviours. Non-verbal skills that come natural to people without impairments need to be taught specifically to people with visual impairments [20], for example by explaining gestures in a tactile way and in natural situations. So even though people with sensory impairments show problems in expressing themselves non-verbally, Gense and Gense [20] do believe that many behaviours can be taught. On the other hand, in visually impaired people some behaviours may be impossible to teach. Making eye contact and following gaze direction are simply infeasible for people with visual impairments. One cannot expect them to show these behaviours. Since their impairments make some social behaviours impossible to execute, they may use other signs to show their social skills. A blind person will not look someone in the eye when interested in what they have to say, but they may aim their ears towards this person and will thus aim their face in another direction. This behaviour is inappropriate for someone with adequate visual abilities, but the visually impaired will orient with their ears more than with their eyes and it may even point to social interest in another person.

Another complication is that it is important to take into account the severity of intellectual disability when analysing a person's social behaviours. If mental and chronological age do not match, age inappropriate social behaviours might be seen. An example is that people with intellectual disabilities show few gestures and joint attention signs [26]. On the other hand, people with mental retardation and autism responded to their name much less frequently than did people with mental retardation alone [26], making orientation after hearing ones name a characteristic that may help in differentiating autistic from non-autistic people.

When trying to differentiate autistic behaviours from behaviours due to multiple impairments, Hoevenaars-van den Boom et al. (2009) showed that even though social behaviours appear similar it is possible to differentiate autistic from non-autistic behaviours. They have found a significant difference between autistic and non-autistic deafblind children with profound intellectual disabilities in the areas of social and communicative behaviours in that these children showed and openness for contact and pleasure while in social contact [7].

2.3. Joint attention and theory of mind

Autistic people have trouble sharing interests, emotions and activities [2]. Related to this is problems in joint attention. Joint attention refers to the ability to share your attention, by looking where someone else is looking at and by sharing your own interests through pointing, gazing, or other non-verbal behaviour [19]. People with ASD may fail to share their emotions, feelings and thoughts but they also can have problems in sharing attention, which is expressed in their inability to follow a pointing finger or the direction of a gaze. This is interesting, because in non-autistic children, both pointing and following a finger or gaze not only relates to the object itself, but also to the other person's feelings and interests for this object. Autistic people fail to point or gaze and follow somebody else's pointing or gazing because they fail to understand other people's interests in the objects [19].

Joint attention is often said to be a precursor of theory of mind (ToM) [27]. Someone has a ToM when they are capable of attributing a mental state to themselves and to others [28]. ToM is one of the most important constructs regarding a deeper understanding of ASD [29] and can explain many of the symptoms of ASD. Not only social behaviours as joint attention, but also symbolic play and language problems such as echolalia and reversal of pronouns can be attributed to not having a ToM [12, 30]. In simple terms, its refers to being able to realize what people think, feel and want [3]. Having a ToM also entails understanding irony and non-literal language, and can therefore also explain some of the deficits in communication. Another aspect of ToM is being able to take someone else's point of view or perspective. Perspective taking is often measured with false belief tasks, such as the Sally-Anne-task [31]. Baron-Cohen and colleagues used this task to measure false belief in autistic children by showing them two dolls, one called Sally and the other called Anne. They played out a story where Sally had a marble in her basket. Sally left and Anne put the marble in her own basket. By asking children questions on where the marble really is and where Sally would think the marble is, perspective taking can be measured [32] and give an indication of the development of a ToM. This is a typical false belief task, but many variations have been used since then. Where in sighted children ToM is tested with a false belief task such as the Sally-Anne task [32] or joint attention tasks, these tasks may not be applicable sufficiently enough for children with visual impairment. In addition, joint attention is often measured with gaze direction or pointing, something that blind children are for obvious reasons incapable of showing and is limited in visually impaired children. Peréz-Pereira and Conti-Ramsden do point out that it is not the pointing or gazing what matters, it is the function of this pointing that is of interest [30]. To measure this, things need to be seen from a blind person's perspective.

Seeing things from a blind person's perspective is difficult when it comes to ToM tasks. Conventional ToM tasks have been carried out on people with impaired vision, showing that visually impaired children invariably performed worse than sighted children. McAlpine and Moore did a false belief task using containers with unexpected contents and asked what another person would think was in it. Many of the blind children failed this task, even though sighted children are able to do this at a younger age [33, 34]. A similar study by Minter, Hobson and Bishop (1998) compared visually impaired with sighted children of the same verbal intelligence, and showed similar results. In their first experiment, they did a similar task as the container task McAlpine and Moore used. They used a warm teapot, filled with sand instead of tea. Whereas almost all sighted children were able to pass this task, almost half of the visually impaired children failed to answer false belief questions such as: "What did you think was in here?" and "What would he/she think is in here?" The authors note that blind people may have less experience with hot teapots because of the extra danger their lack of vision provides. Their second experiment was done with three boxes, where the participants helped the experimenter hide a pencil for another experimenter and false belief questions were asked. Again, the visually impaired children performed worse than the sighted, but much better than on the previous task. The authors think this was because they were more involved in this task, because they helped with the hiding [35]. These findings show that children with visual impairments do worse on conventional ToM tasks than do their hearing peers. One could assume that blind children do not have a ToM, or develop it slower. However, other findings indicate that visually impaired children can pass a ToM task, given an adapted task. In line with the notion that things need to be seen more from a blind person's perspective, it could be possible that visually impaired people have just as much a ToM as sighted people do; it's only measured in the wrong way. Peterson and her colleagues confirmed this. They state that blind people may very well rely on completely different features of an object than sighted people do in order to decide what another person thinks about an object [36]. They tested if this was true by adapting frequently used false belief tasks. For example, they have changed the famous Sally-Anne task to a Sally-Bill task. In this task, there were no dolls or pictures of children with baskets and marbles, but it was a purely narrative story. The experimenters performed four ToM tasks, including similar tasks to the container tasks, a location change task and a story. On average, the children performed best on the Sally-Bill task, 73% of the children passed this task. Despite this result and the careful adaptation of test methods, test methods were not found to be a factor influencing ToM development. Degree of visual impairment was also not found to be of influence in developing a ToM, age was the only significant factor these authors found [36]. These are some interesting findings, firstly because they indicate that visually impaired people can show signs of having a ToM, secondly, because the question is raised where the difference lies between visually impaired and sighted people. According to Minter et al. [35] tasks need to be adapted to the qualities of visually impaired but Peterson et al. [37] did not find a difference between tasks they used. Brambring and Ashbrock [38] elaborated on this question. They used a large variety of different tasks that did not require vision and found that performance was better than with traditional tasks but the blind children were on average 19 months older when they were able to perform the same tasks as sighted children. A more recent study [39] found that children with varying levels of congenital visual impairment when compared with sighted children matched on age and verbal intelligence, had a similar performance on advanced ToM stories (second order false belief, that is beliefs about beliefs) and non-literal stories. Despite a limited access to visual information during interactions, children with congenital visual impairment can develop an effective ToM.

Peterson has not only studied ToM in visually impaired children, but also in deaf children [37, 40]. It looks as if deaf children are strongly delayed or even impaired in their ability to have a ToM. In their 1995 study, Peterson and Siegal tested the Sally-Anne paradigm on several deaf children who were able to communicate in sign language. Even though hearing children with or without intellectual disabilities can pass this task around a mental age of four, only 35% of these deaf children were able to pass at a mental age of 8. Furthermore, these results were similar to results of people with ASD, but worse than the performance of children with Down syndrome. Notwithstanding the lack of ToM, these deaf children were not autistic as they did not show any of the other characteristics of ASD [40]. According to Peterson and Siegel deaf children lack a ToM, because of the lack of understanding the communicative signals of others. It also appears that deaf children, especially those with hearing parents, communicate less at home than hearing children. On the one hand this is because a deaf child does not hear nor understand spoken language and on the other hand because their parents are not very fluent in sign language as an alternative for spoken language [41]. A direct consequence of the lower frequency of communication is that deaf children also communicate less about mental states, feelings and thoughts, which hinders the development of a ToM [37, 40]. This idea was supported in a more recent study that assessed the amount of communication in play sessions for pairs of hearing mothers with their deaf children and compared them to hearing mothers with hearing children. They found that these signing mothers of deaf children do not necessarily communicate less than mothers of hearing children, but they do communicate less about mental states. Additionally, a relationship was found between the amount of communication about mental states of mothers of deaf children and the performance on false belief tasks of their children [42]. Despite the similar way in which the lack of ToM expresses itself in people with ASD and in deaf, the cause is different. In children who are deaf it is often attributed to a lack of communication about mental states, thoughts and feelings, whereas in ASD it is caused by inability to take someone else's perspective.

Another possibility for why hearing children outperform deaf children on ToM tasks could be that deaf children do have a ToM but only fail on certain aspects related to ToM and conventional tasks fail to test these aspects. Where normally false belief tests and variations of this are undertaken, a recent study addressed other aspects of ToM as well. Ketelaar, Rieffe, Wiefferink and Frijns [43] assessed deaf children that have received a cochlear implant (CI) at a young age, and compared them to hearing children. They tested other aspects of ToM than false belief, which are the understanding of other's intentions and others desires. The tasks were similar to false belief tasks, only instead of asking what someone would think or believe, it was asked what an other person intended to do with an object (after failing this action) or what someone would want to eat (after showing them pictures of food they liked). It appeared that the deaf children and hearing children performed equally well on the intention tasks, but the hearing children outperformed the deaf on false belief tasks and on the desire tasks [43].This study indicates that deaf children may possess some abilities related to a theory of mind. It should be noted, however, that this study only included children with a CI. These children thus had some hearing abilities, though different from hearing children. The study did not include a group that was completely deaf and so conclusions about completely deaf children cannot be drawn.

When children are completely deaf there is, however, still the possibility that, as seen in the visually impaired group, testing methods are not adequate for them. Peterson and Siegal [40] tried to make their intentions more clear in their false belief questions. They reasoned that someone with limited experience in conversation might expect that the experimenter just wants them to tell the location of Sally's marble, when they ask "Where will Sally look for her marble?" For this reason they altered the question to "Where will Sally first look for her marble?" By adding the word "first" they more clearly imply that they are looking for what sally thinks instead of where the marble really is. This slight alteration improved the deaf children's performance slightly, but not enough to overcome differences in ToM development [40] as the different tasks in the study by Ketalaar et al. [43] did. Peterson and Siegal only investigated false belief, though, whereas Ketelaar et al. adressesd other aspects of ToM and tested children with a CI who do have some hearing abilities, instead of children who are completely unable to hear. The question still remains whether a more appropriate methodology for deaf children could increase their scores on conventional ToM tasks and more research has to be done in order to clarify this.

Finally, people with intellectual disabilities often show ToM impairments as well. Typical developing children start to solve ToM tasks around the age of four to five years of age. A general characteristic of people with intellectual disabilities is that they have mental ages not corresponding to their chronological ages. If mental age is below five, which is the case in profoundly and severely intellectually disabled people, and sometimes also in moderately intellectually impaired people they will probably fail ToM tasks irrespective of their chronological age [44]. Interpretations of ToM tasks should be done cautiously, when intellectually disabled people likely fail this task unrelated to the presence of ASD, to prevent unnecessary suspicion of ASD.

3. Qualitative impairments in communication

Qualitative impairments in communication form the second criterion that is defined in DSM-IV-TR, and this can refer to the use of language but also to problems in make belief or imitative play. When it comes to language one can find a lack of or delay in language, but also use of repetitive or idiosyncratic language. Autistic people may also find it troubling to initiate and maintain a conversation with others [2].

3.1. Making conversation

Language is something people use for communication, and so the willingness to communicate is related to their use of language [19].Despite possible technical problems in language
the low desire for communication is one of the aspects of ASD that is mentioned in the
DSM-IV-TR, that is not only problems in initiating and maintaining a conversation with others but also a lack of an internal willingness or desire to communicate [2]. If people with
ASD are simply uninterested in communication, they will not put effort in initiating a social
conversation spontaneously. This lack in willingness to communicate also contributes to the
language problems found in ASD.

Initiating and maintaining a conversation can be difficult for people with sensory and intellectual disabilities too. The presence of others may go unnoticed for people with visual impairments, and communicative signs may be missed because of blindness or deafness. It has
been found that deaf children communicate less with their hearing parents because of their
poor skills in spoken language and their parents poor sign language skills [41]. In people
with intellectual disabilities conversational skills may be worse than expected based on their
chronological age, moreover, their initiations to communicate may be different, inadequate
or even awkward.

Even though all of these impaired groups may show impaired conversation making skills,
there are differences between autistic and non-autistic people. An example derived from a
deaf population shows that despite other problems in the field of communication, such as
monitoring a conversation and pragmatic use of language, non-autistic deaf children are not
different from their hearing peers in initiating and maintaining a conversation [22]. But even
though deaf children without ASD don't seem to have problems in initiating and maintaining a conversation, they still differ from their hearing peers in pragmatics and monitoring,
hampering their conversational skills nevertheless. On the contrary, the impaired conversational skills in autistic people lie in the area of the initiation and maintenance of a conversation [2]. It also appeared that one of the areas in which the autistic and non-autistic children
with deafblindness and profound intellectual disability differed significantly from each other was the openness and willingness to take initiatives for contact [7]. It is evident that conversation looks different for people with sensory or intellectual impairments versus people
without impairments, and conversation skills are hampered by their lack of sensory and intellectual abilities. The difference with autistic people shows itself in the interest for this contact. Non-autistic sensory and/or intellectually impaired people still look for opportunities
to make this contact or respond to other people's efforts to make contact, while people with
autism lack the interest for this contact.

3.2. Language

Besides a lower interest in communication than people without ASD, people with ASD
show some technical language impairments as well. Some autistic people do not speak at all
and in others the development of language can be seriously delayed or altered [19]. Furthermore, it appears that joint attention and imitation behaviours, which are known to be impaired in ASD, can predict language abilities [27], which raises the question whether

language is directly or indirectly related to ASD. In addition, ToM can be involved as well, one needs to know that one can influence others with their language and how to do so. Typical ASD language problems include direct or delayed echolalia, reversal of pronouns and lack of understanding of emotional meaning in language. People often describe it as 'robot-like' [45]. People with ASD often interpret the meaning of words literally. The literal meaning of a word does not change over contexts, but the figural meaning does. This is especially vivid in jokes, metaphors and irony. This may also be due to the previously mentioned problems in ToM. Being unable to understand what people mean, people with ASD interpret the words incorrectly [19]. A review about language and communication in ASD confirmed this idea by concluding that the language and communication problems are caused by processing problems when interacting with other people [46].

People with intellectual disabilities show delays in language as well as atypical language skills that can easily be confused with ASD. A study about the language abilities of a group of autistic children showed that there was a relationship between language abilities and IQ [46]. This study was done on autistic people only, but it is a rather expectable finding, even within people without ASD. It makes sense that the language abilities of someone with an intellectual disability are delayed as compared to peers with the same chronological age. This may be confused with the language deficits found in ASD, when in fact they are due to their intellectual disability. For this reason, we should not immediately attribute language issues in people with intellectual disabilities to ASD.

Deaf and people with hearing disabilities often show delays in acquiring language, but can also show peculiar uses of words [4]. Even delays in developing sign language are found for this is often not fully learned until children go to a school for the deaf. Parents are not fluent signers and fail to teach children the full scope of signs they could learn from a signer that is fluent [41]. Atypical language development can also be found in the blind. Without seeing things to potentially talk about, language is centred around other experiences in the blind compared to sighted people [18]. Children with congenital visual impairment have been shown to have difficulties with the use of language for pragmatic and social purposes, while structural language (e.g. articulation, grammar, vocabulary) was good or even superior [47, 48]. This delay or odd language use can be confused with what is found in autistic individuals. However, this language delay may be corrected if it is taught in the right way. It's important to realise that when a child misses its vision, they need to get stimulation through the other senses which affects their understanding of the meaning of words [18].

Several language problems that are found in autistic individuals are also found in people with other impairments. A typical example is echolalia, which is also found in visually and intellectually impaired people [23]. Echolalia is the apparently useless repeating of words or phrases, either immediately after they were spoken or after some time. Even in typically developing children, echolalia is sometimes used to learn language [20], so it's not surprising to find this in people with intellectual disabilities who may have a mental age comparable to when it is normal to use this type of speech. According to Schlesinger, it can be expected for a typically developing 20 month year old to repeat words to indicate more than one (e.g. "apple, apple" for "two apples") [49]. Another author described a child of 15 – 18 months old who often repeated her mother's words to learn the names of objects, but also to practice these words [50]. It can therefore be expected that a person with a mental age below two years of age to still show signs of echolalia. These examples consist of people with typically developing vision, but blind children use echolalia even more than typically developing children. In part echolalia serves as a means to stay in contact with people that cannot be seen, but it is also suggested that blind children practice their language by using echolalic speech. In this way they try to get a grip on the meaning of words in the absence of vision [30]. Extra practicing of words and phrases also results in more imitations and use of routines in speech. In the blind, one will also find egocentric speech and reversal of personal pronouns(I, you, he etc.), and improper use of deictic terms (e.g. here, there) which could be mistaken for autistic language, because of its atypical nature. Reversal of personal pronouns, which is found in about a third of the speech of blind children and egocentric speech may be caused by a lack of ToM, resulting in these impairments [12]. However, a logical explanation can also be based on the visual impairment. The direction of speech and who is speaking to whom determines which personal pronoun is used. Absence of vision makes it difficult to understand that the "I" who is speaking about the self is suddenly referred to as "you" by a person who became the "I" instead. 'Here' and 'there' are relative terms depending on ones spatial position. Without sight it is hard to adopt an allocentric position, most blind people use an egocentric position in processing spatial information. For instance, in way finding one cannot use landmark information to guide people who are blind, because they cannot see these landmarks. Instead one has to give route information related to the blind person's body position in space [30].

3.3. Imitation and make-belief or symbolic play

Finally, imitative and make-belief play are impaired in people with ASD according to the DSM-IV-TR. People with intellectually disabilities normally show delays or absence of imitation too. In one study, the experimenters showed intellectually disabled participants an action that could be done with an object, afterwards they asked the participants what could be done with the object. All participants with intellectual disabilities had trouble recalling what could be done with the object. Participants with intellectual disability and ASD performed the worst [51].

Symbolic play can be troubled in people with intellectual disabilities as well. Wing and colleagues [52] showed that even though only two people of their sample of intellectually disabled people showed the full autistic syndrome, more than half of their participants showed problems in symbolic play. These problems were either characterized as stereotyped play that was a persevering repetitive copy of other's play or no symbolic play at all, but just repetitive manipulations of a part of an object. Despite the fact that only two of their participants had an ASD diagnosis, many showed autistic features. In the group that was able to show symbolic play (43 of 108 participants), only two participants had slight autistic features [52].This finding shows that many intellectual disabled people show impairments in symbolic or make-belief play, and this can therefore not be used as a differentiating characteristic of ASD versus no ASD in this group.

When these people with intellectual disabilities have an additional sensory impairment, problems in symbolic play and imitation can become more evident. It is reasonable to think that people with impaired vision or hearing have more difficulties in imitating because they are less able to perceive actions of others, than people without these impairments. Similarly, symbolic play can be affected. People have less modalities to perceive a toy with, and therefore also see less ways in which they may use it. Combined with an intellectual impairment they can also have troubles in understanding the function the object is intended to have.

Lack of symbolic play was demonstrated to be related to abnormalities in language development that are typical of ASD, such as repetitive speech [52]. Similar to many of the impairments in ASD that were discussed, this too can be attributed to a lack of ToM. According to Brown et al. [12] ASD is characterized by problems in ToM, symbolic play, and context dependent language. Shared features of these three skills in childhood are: 1) there has to be a communication pattern between parent and child regarding feelings and thoughts; 2) one has to see and understand the direction of someone else's attitudes towards a shared world; and 3) feel inclined to identify oneself with this shared world. People with ASD have problems with all three features. Children who are deaf encounter problems with the first feature. They are offered less ToM related language. Children who are blind have trouble with the second feature and subsequently children who are deafblind have trouble with the first and second feature.

4. Restricted, repetitive and stereotyped patterns of behaviour

As the last of three important characteristics, the DSM-IV-TR mentions restricted, repetitive and stereotyped patterns of behaviour, interests and activities. This can refer to motoric stereotypies or mannerisms, preoccupations with objects, parts of objects or interests, or their inflexibility in deviating from routines [2].

4.1. Stereotyped use of objects

Uta Frith confirms that autistic people are often very interested in details, which may appear as restricted interests to others [3] and that routines and repetitions are also of importance for them [19].These behaviour can be explained by the central coherence theory. This theory poses that autistic people have a weak central coherence, meaning that they have the tendency perceive objects and situations in parts rather than perceiving the whole picture or combine information to holistic patterns [3]. As a consequence information is often processed out of context [31]. This theory explains the focus on details, but possibly also the need for repetition and routines shown by people with ASD. The ability to generalize parts to the whole keeps situations similar and predictable, and therefore less frightening. If one misses this ability then a coping mechanism is to stick to routines in order to keep situations predictable and safe. If preformed to the extreme these routines become stereotyped behaviours.

Repetitive and stereotyped use of objects is not only seen in autistic people but also in people with intellectual disabilities. In a study where 108 children with severe and profound mental disabilities were included less than two percent suffered from ASD. However, repetitive routines and stereotyped play were found in 60 percent of this group with a mental age below 20 months [52]. Also in children who are blind strong interest in parts of objects and repetitive use of objects can be seen. Mainly this is the result of the blindness-specific constraints on the use of play material that require visual-manual skills. Blind children, when playing alone, prefer toys and materials that produce distinctive tactile or auditory effects [53]. Toys are often articles of daily living and objects in their surroundings such as spoons, walls and furniture. Activities are often aimed at making noise [53, 54].This behaviour is thought to be a way of getting hold on the function of an object and in contrast to children with ASD this behaviour can be relatively easily stopped or interrupted.

4.2. Self Stimulation

Finally, autistic people show stereotyped movements with their own bodies or parts of their body. These are often thought to be self-stimulatory. Stereotyped movements can be performed with every body part but often involve the hands or walking [55, 56] and sometimes become self-injurious [57, 58]. These movements occur in other developmental disorders as well [55, 56], but are especially common in ASD. According to Kraijer self-stimulatory behaviours are often caused by lack of stimulation from the environment [44]. In these situations people use their own bodies to provide themselves with the stimulation they need at that moment. He adds to this that the amount of self-stimulatory behaviour and also intensity and severity, that is whether it is self-injurious, is related to the level of functioning. The lower the functional level of the person, the more the self-stimulatory behaviour increases in amount and severity [44].

Stereotyped behaviours occur in people with visual impairments as well. Typical stereotyped behaviours in people who are blind are body rocking, head shaking, eye poking and hand flapping Because these behaviours often occur in the blind, they are sometimes referred to as blindisms, [18, 20]. Actually this term is not entirely correct, because these stereotyped behaviours are not unique for people who are blind; mannerisms would be a better term. Body rocking and head movements, for instance, are typical examples of behaviours that can be seen in people with visual impairment, intellectual disabilities and ASD [18, 20, 24]. Stereotyped behaviours were seen in nearly all [59] and in all [60] blind children, but in children with visual impairment the prevalence is still 10-45% [59]. There also seems to be an age dependency in stereotyped behaviours in blind children. In the first two years stereotyped behaviours increase in frequency to decline thereafter [61]. Stereotyped movements are also found in people with multiple disabilities. Heather Murdoch [62] suggests that stereotyped behaviours may be a part of normal motor development but that in people with multiple disabilities, these behaviours do not develop further. In a typically developing child, repetitive behaviours appear as well but develop into conscious movements later on, whereas in people with multiple disabilities they may remain repetitive movements. Trying to stop these behaviours may hamper the development of other motor activities or communicative signs [62].

Whereas stereotyped movements in people without ASD are part of a normal development, in people with ASD they are part of their syndrome. Gense and Gense [20] believe that the differences between these behaviours in visually impaired people with or without ASD can be found in the severity and perseverance of this behaviour. People with ASD show higher intensities and stronger persistence in stereotypical behaviours [20, 57]. Similar to the behaviours in the intellectually disabled, this could be due to a lack of external stimulation. Especially in the blind, where stimulation from visual input is missing, self-stimulatory stereotyped movements could provide the necessary sensory stimulation [18]. Another difference between people with ASD and people without, is that stereotyped behaviour can more easily be interrupted or stopped in people with visual impairments alone [20]. Sometimes not much more has to be undertaken than making the blind person conscious of these unconsciously executed stereotyped behaviour patterns.

5. Differentiation: Why and how?

5.1. Overlap and differences

The overlap in symptoms between autistic and non-autistic people with sensory and intellectual disabilities must be clear after reading this chapter. The diagnoses of ASD is usually based on behavioural characteristics and these can be similar in autistic and non-autistic people with additional impairments. An additional problem is that, although instruments are available for people with intellectual disabilities [63, 64], most of the current test instruments do not have separate norms for people with sensory and/or intellectual disabilities. No valid instruments are available for deaf people according to Jure and colleagues [14], nor for visually impaired people [7]. The overlap in symptoms and trouble in diagnosis cause a distorted representation of ASD in people with sensory, intellectual and multiple impairments. Some people are diagnosed as autistic when they are not, while others do not get the autistic label when they should. So there is both an overdiagnosis [5, 15] of ASD in this group, meaning that more people are diagnosed as autistic than necessary because of these overlapping symptoms, as well as an underdiagnosis [14, 65]. In a group of deaf children, for example, the diagnosis of ASD was established significantly later than in a group of hearing children. Autistic behaviours were probably missed because of an earlier diagnosis of hearing impairments or other developmental disabilities [65]. The main problem in assessment of ASD can be attributed to a diagnostic overshadowing bias. The diagnostic overshadowing bias was first described for people with intellectual disabilities and is the tendency of clinicians to overlook symptoms of mental health problems in this group and attribute them to being part of "having an intellectual disability" [66]. In the presence of mental retardation it seems that the diagnostic importance of abnormal behaviour decreases. Blindness, deafness or deafblindness all might add an extra overshadowing bias next to intellectual disability, leading to either false positive or false negative diagnoses of ASD in people with these disabilities.

Despite the obvious similarities between autistic and non-autistic people with sensory and intellectual disabilities, this chapter also outlines that even though the symptoms appear the same, sometimes subtle difference can still be found. This may be due to the possibility that underlying processes of the behaviours are different for autistic and non-autistic individuals [4, 5, 15]. If attempted, a differentiation can thus be made by studying the subtle differences and underlying causes. A couple of years ago, this was done by making a valid instrument to diagnose ASD in people one of the most challenging combination of disabilities, namely deafblindness and profound intellectual disabilities. Hoevenaars-van den Boom and colleagues were able to confirm the huge overlap in behavioural symptoms between autistic and non-autistic people, but were also able to successfully distinguish the autistic from non-autistic people with their approach that was suited to the developmental level of the participants. They found that differences in this group can be found in the social communicative field, mostly in openness for contact, reciprocity and joint attention and communicative functions [7]. It is clear that when using a careful and sophisticated approach, a distinction can be made between autistic and non-autistic people with sensory and intellectual disabilities

5.2. Interaction, treatment and teaching

A fair diagnosis of ASD, or no ASD, is very important for the treatment and interaction with people with sensory and intellectual disabilities. An ASD diagnosis or a lack thereof will affect how a person will be treated, as autistic or not. If a child with ASD is placed in a setting where his or her ASD goes unrecognized, the clinicians and care takers might fail to respond to the needs of this person [65]. An important example of why recognition of ASD is so important is the treatment of stereotyped behaviour. Stereotyped movements can be a way to reduce stress [19, 20]. In someone with no ASD but with blindness or deafblindness, this behaviour is usually caused when the person does not get enough stimulation from their environment [17, 18], whereas in persons with ASD stereotyped behaviours can be a way to escape from overstimulation or as a way to ensure the optimal level of arousal. In both cases the way to treat stereotyped behaviour will be different, give extra stimulation or reduce overstimulation, respectively. A valid diagnosis would be very helpful in cases where clinicians or parents have to decide what kind of intervention to give. If it is clear whether someone has ASD or not treatment and interaction can be adjusted. Someone with ASD needs a more structured environment, and needs clear instructions when something needs to be done. In someone with ASD, things need to be re-explained in new situations, because of their difficulties in generalizing [6]. It also seems that the sooner we are aware of ASD the better. People with ASD need to be approached in way that is accommodated to their needs [65], and for the wellbeing of the child, it is best if this is done as soon as possible. A recent meta-analysis on intensive early intervention programs for ASD shows that programs that intervene early are most effective and can produce changes in the area of language and adaptive behaviour [67]. Adaptive behaviour was also found to increase as well when additional behavioural treatments were given to children with ASD and intellectual disabilities [68]. These studies showed that if ASD is treated, successful results can be achieved.

As can be seen throughout this chapter, people with visual impairments show many behaviours that are similar to ASD, such as the lack of understanding of social situations, ego-centeredness, and lack of understanding gestures and facial expressions. But, according to Gense and Gense [20], these behaviours may still be taught. Teaching appropriate behaviours is especially important, because inappropriate behaviours may interfere with regular social interactions [18], depriving disabled children of these otherwise valuable experiences. And whereas for non-autistic people without visual impairments these behaviours are implicitly learned, in non-autistic visually impaired people, they need to be explicitly taught. With the right type of education, visually impaired people may still learn to interpret social situations, read and understand gestures and facial expressions and learn to play with others [20]. This was also found for two severely mentally disabled deafblind young men, of whom the social interaction became significantly better after tailored training sessions [58]. Although this was only a small study with two participants, it does indicate what a specialized training can mean for children that are not restrained by ASD. The same applies to language. When a delay in language is caused by a lack of seeing things to talk about, parents need to offer more tactile or auditory stimuli [18]. Basically, it is important to take into account everything that singular or multiple disabled people lack. When sensory and intellectual impairments are involved, one needs to try and substitute the missing modality for others as much as possible.

6. Summary and Conclusion

Many characteristics of ASD seem to overlap with characteristics that are naturally present in people with sensory disabilities, intellectual impairments or a combination of disabilities. The characteristics appear the same whether ASD is present or not, which makes it difficult to make a valid diagnosis of ASD in this group. All of the criteria that are used in DSM-IV-TR to define ASD are, to some extent, also present in people with one or more of these disabilities. However, if one would look closer to these criteria, and the way they are expressed within people with sensory and intellectual impairments, slight and subtle differences can be found. There are differences in the way the symptoms express themselves, the severity of the symptoms and the underlying causes for the behaviours. Problems also occur in methodology. Paradigms that are used to assess problems that are related to ASD, such as ToM tasks, fail to be successful in differentiating people with sensory or multiple impairments. This overlap and these problems in methodology make it a major challenge to diagnose ASD within people with sensory and intellectual disabilities.

The slight differences in the way symptoms are expressed show that a distinction between autistic behaviours and non-autistic behaviours can be made. Making this distinction is very important to do, because the needs of people with ASD differ very much from people without ASD. To make sure the needs of every individual are met, people should be diagnosed in the right way. This is especially important for those groups with problems in communicating their wants and needs. In order to do this, subtle differences need to be taken into account. Up until this day, no instrument is suited to diagnose ASD or assess autistic behaviours within multiply impaired people. Ideally, a new way to assess autistic behaviours in sensory and intellectually disabled people that takes into account all the difficulties that assessing this group brings forth will be developed. An instrument that can make accurate diagnosis in people with multiple disabilities should account for all the overlapping symptoms and differences that have been described. First of all, intellectual disabilities should be taken into account. Some behaviours that are typical for ASD in people without intellectual disabilities can be simply explained by a person's mental age or shortcomings in intellectual abilities. An example of this is theory of mind, and related to that joint attention, symbolic play and language abilities, that do not develop until a certain age. If an intellectually disabled person has not reached a sufficient mental age, these behaviours should not be used to assess ASD. Secondly, it's important to realise that sensory disabilities withhold a person from perceiving objects and situations the same way a person without sensory disabilities would and may follow a completely different path. When someone is visually impaired or blind, eye contact, following gaze and sharing attention through pointing cannot be used as differentiating characteristics. Furthermore, it's important to take into account that a person may not always be aware of the presence of objects or people, so failures to respond like a person without ASD can be caused by being unaware of their presence in the first place. Similar precautions should be made for deaf people, who are unable to respond to calling their names, other sounds, and may not even notice the arrival or departure of a person. Finally, a combination of these disabilities can make it more challenging to make diagnostic evaluations of a person. People with multiple disabilities may need more time to process their surroundings and to realise what is expected of them. Furthermore, unexpected and sudden movements or actions, or giving too much information at once may cause a lot of stress that interferes with their performance. Many characteristics that normally differentiate people with ASD from people without ASD should not be assessed or assessed differently in people with multiple impairments. Still, some characteristics of the autistic spectrum are left that can be included in an assessment. Examples that cannot be forgotten include interest in, response to and looking for contact, resistance to change and interest in new items or situations. Sharing of feelings or interests may not occur through pointing or gaze, but may show itself in a more tactile way. It is important to be aware of the different way in which multiply disabled people express themselves. Finally, to account for intellectual disabilities, it is important to assess everything on a level that is suitable for the participants. Do not use complicated questionnaires, but simple toys as much as possible. Only if all of this can be done successfully, autistic people can be differentiated from non-autistic people and personal needs can be met.

Author details

Gitta De Vaan[1*], Mathijs P.J. Vervloed[1], Harry Knoors[1,2] and Ludo Verhoeven[1]

*Address all correspondence to: g.devaan@pwo.ru.nl

1 Behavioural Science Institute, Radboud University Nijmegen, NijmegenThe Netherlands,

2 Royal Kentalis, Sint-Michielsgestel, The Netherlands

References

[1] Nevid JS, Rathus SA, Greene B. Abnormal psychology in a changing world. 7th ed. Upper Saddle River, NJ: Pearson Education; 2008.

[2] American Psychiatric Association. Diagnostic and statistical manual of mental disorders, fourth edition, text revision (DSM-IV-TR). Washington, DC: American Psychiatric Association; 2000.

[3] Frith U. Autism: A very short introduction. Oxford, United Kingdom: Oxford University Press; 2008.

[4] Knoors H, Vervloed MPJ. Educational programming for deaf children with multiple disabilities: Accomodating special needs. In: Marschark M, Spencer PE, editors. The Oxford Handbook of Deaf Studies, Language and Education. 2 ed. New York: Oxford University Press; 2011. p. 82-96.

[5] Cass H. Visual Impairment and Autism. Autism. 1998 June 1, 1998;2(2):117-38.

[6] De Bildt A, Sytema S, Kraijer D, Minderaa R. Prevalence of pervasive developmental disorders in children and adolescents with mental retardation. Journal of Child Psychology and Psychiatry. 2005;46(3):275-86.

[7] Hoevenaars-van den Boom MAA, Antonissen ACFM, Knoors H, Vervloed MPJ. Differentiating characteristics of deafblindness and autism in people with congenital deafblindness and profound intellectual disability. Journal of Intellectual Disability Research. 2009;53(6):548-58.

[8] Fombonne E. The prevalence of autism. JAMA: The Journal of the American Medical Association. 2003;289(1):87-9.

[9] Fombonne E. Epidemiological Surveys of Autism and Other Pervasive Developmental Disorders: An Update. Journal of Autism and Developmental Disorders. 2003;33(4):365-82.

[10] Kim YS, Leventhal BL, Koh Y-J, Fombonne E, Laska E, Lim E-C, et al. Prevalence of Autism Spectrum Disorders in a Total Population Sample. American Journal of Psychiatry. 2011;168:904-12.

[11] Matson JL, Shoemaker M. Intellectual disability and its relationship to autism spectrum disorders. Research in Developmental Disabilities. 2009;30(6):1107-14.

[12] Brown R, Hobson RP, Lee A, Stevenson J. Are There "Autistic-like" Features in Congenitally Blind Children? Journal of Child Psychology and Psychiatry. 1997;38(6): 693-703.

[13] Hobson RP, Lee A, Brown R. Autism and Congenital Blindness. Journal of Autism and Developmental Disorders. 1999;29(1):45-56.

[14] Jure R, Rapin I, Tuchman RF. Hearing-impaired autistic children. Developmental Medicine & Child Neurology. 1991;33(12):1062-72.

[15] Andrews R, Wyver S. Autistic tendencies: Are there different pathways for blindness and Autism Spectrum Disorder? British Journal of Visual Impairment. 2005 May 1, 2005;23(2):52-7.

[16] Hobson RP. Why connect? On the relation between autism and blindness. In: Pring L, editor. Autism and Blindness: Research and reflections. London, United Kingdom: Whurr Publishers; 2005. p. 10-25.

[17] Van Dijk J, Janssen M. Doofblinde kinderen [Deafblind children]. In: Nakken H, editor. Meervoudig gehandicapten: een zorg apart. Rotterdam, the Netherlands: Lemniscaat; 1993.

[18] Warren DH. Blindness and Children: An individual differences approach. Cambridge, UK: Cambridge University Press; 1994.

[19] Frith U. Autism: Explaining the enigma. 2nd ed. Oxford, UK: Blackwell Publishing; 2003.

[20] Gense MH, Gense DJ. Autism Spectrum Disorders and Visual Impairment: Meeting Student's Learning Needs. New York, NY: American Foundation for the Blind Press; 2005.

[21] Baranek GT. Autism During Infancy: A Retrospective Video Analysis of Sensory-Motor and Social Behaviors at 9–12 Months of Age. Journal of Autism and Developmental Disorders. 1999;29(3):213-24.

[22] Wolters N, Knoors HET, Cillessen AHN, Verhoeven L. Predicting acceptance and popularity in early adolescence as a function of hearing status, gender, and educational setting. Research in Developmental Disabilities. 2011;32(6):2553-65.

[23] Wing L, Gould J. Severe impairments of social interaction and associated abnormalities in children: Epidemiology and classification. Journal of Autism and Developmental Disorders. 1979;9(1):11-29.

[24] Fraiberg S. Insights from the blind. New York, NY: Basic Books; 1977.

[25] Ainsworth MDS, Bell SM. Attachment, Exploration, and Separation: Illustrated by the Behavior of One-Year-Olds in a Strange Situation. Child Development. 1970;41(1):49-67.

[26] Osterling JA, Dawson G, Munson JA. Early recognition of 1-year-old infants with autism spectrum disorder versus mental retardation. Development and Psychopathology. 2002;14(02):239-51.

[27] Charman T, Baron-Cohen S, Swettenham J, Baird G, Cox A, Drew A. Testing joint attention, imitation, and play as infancy precursors to language and theory of mind. Cognitive Development. 2000;15(4):481-98.

[28] Premack D, Woodruff G. Does the chimpanzee have a theory of mind? Behavioral and Brain Sciences. 1978;1(04):515-26.

[29] Noens I, van Berckelaer-Onnes I. Making Sense in a Fragmentary World. Autism. 2004 June 1, 2004;8(2):197-218.

[30] Pérez-Pereira M, Conti-Ramsden G. Language development and social interaction in blind children. East Sussex, UK: Psychology Press; 1999.

[31] Hill EL, Frith U. Understanding autism: insights from mind and brain. Philosophical Transactions of the Royal Society of London Series B: Biological Sciences. 2003 February 28, 2003;358(1430):281-9.

[32] Baron-Cohen S, Leslie AM, Frith U. Does the autistic child have a "theory of mind" ? Cognition. 1985;21(1):37-46.

[33] McAlpine LM, Moore CL. The development of social understanding in children with visual impairments. Journal of Visual Impairment & Blindness. 1995;89(4):349-58.

[34] Pérez-Pereira M, Conti-Ramsden G. Do blind children show autistic features? In: Pring L, editor. Autism and blindness: Research and reflections. London, UK: Whurr Publishers; 2005.

[35] Minter M, Hobson RP, Bishop M. Congenital visual impairment and 'theory of mind'. British Journal of Developmental Psychology. 1998;16(2):183-96.

[36] Peterson CC, Peterson JL, Webb J. Factors influencing the development of a theory of mind in blind children. British Journal of Developmental Psychology. 2000;18(3): 431-47.

[37] Peterson CC, Siegal M. Insights into Theory of Mind from Deafness and Autism. Mind & Language. 2000;15(1):123-45.

[38] Brambring M, Asbrock D. Validity of False Belief Tasks in Blind Children. Journal of Autism and Developmental Disorders. 2010;40(12):1471-84.

[39] Pijnacker J, Vervloed M, Steenbergen B. Pragmatic Abilities in Children with Congenital Visual Impairment: An Exploration of Non-literal Language and Advanced Theory of Mind Understanding. Journal of Autism and Developmental Disorders. 1-10.

[40] Peterson CC, Siegal M. Deafness, Conversation and Theory of Mind. Journal of Child Psychology and Psychiatry. 1995;36(3):459-74.

[41] Vaccari C, Marschark M. Communication between Parents and Deaf Children: Implications for Social-emotional Development. Journal of Child Psychology and Psychiatry. 1997;38(7):793-801.

[42] Moeller MP, Schick B. Relations Between Maternal Input and Theory of Mind Understanding in Deaf Children. Child Development. 2006;77(3):751-66.

[43] Ketelaar L, Rieffe C, Wiefferink CH, Frijns JHM. Does Hearing Lead to Understanding? Theory of Mind in Toddlers and Preschoolers With Cochlear Implants. Journal of Pediatric Psychology. 2012 July 29, 2012.

[44] Kraijer D. Handboek autismespectrumstoornissen en verstandelijke beperking [Handbook autism spectrum disorders and intellectual disability]. Lisse, the Netherlands: Harcourt; 2004.

[45] Nederlandse Vereniging voor Psychiatrie. Richtlijn Diagnostiek en behandeling autismespectrumstoornissen bij kinderen en jeugdigen [Guideline diagnostics and treatment of autism spectrum disorders in children and youth] Utrecht, Netherlands: de Tijdstroom; 2009.

[46] Tager-Flusberg H, Paul R, Lord C. Language and Communication in Autism. In: Volkmar FR, Paul R, Klin A, Cohen DJ, editors. Handbook of Autism and Pervasive Developmental Disorders. 3rd ed2005.

[47] James DM, Stojanovik V. Communication skills in blind children: a preliminary investigation. Child: Care, Health and Development. 2007;33(1):4-10.

[48] Tadić V, Pring L, Dale N. Are language and social communication intact in children with congenital visual impairment at school age? Journal of Child Psychology and Psychiatry. 2010;51(6):696-705.

[49] Schlesinger IM. Steps to Language. Toward a theory of native language aquisition. Hillsdale, NJ: Lawrence Erlbaum Associates; 1982.

[50] Dore J. A pragmatic description of early language development. Journal of Psycholinguistic Research. 1974;3(4):343-50.

[51] Charman T, Swettenham J, Baron-Cohen S, Cox A, Baird G, Drew A. Infants with autism: An investigation of empathy, pretend play, joint attention, and imitation. Developmental Psychology. 1997;33(5):781-9.

[52] Wing L, Gould J, Yeates SR, Brierly LM. Symbolic play in severely mentally retared and in autistic children. Journal of Child Psychology and Psychiatry. 1977;18(2): 167-78.

[53] Tröster H, Brambring M. The play behavior and play materials of blind and sighted infants and preschoolers. Journal of Visual Impairment & Blindness. 1994;88(5): 421-32.

[54] Preisler GM. A descriptive study of blind children in nurseries with sighted children. Child: Care, Health and Development. 1993;19(5):295-315.

[55] Goldman S, Wang C, Salgado MW, Greene PE, Kim M, Rapin I. Motor stereotypies in children with autism and other developmental disorders. Developmental Medicine & Child Neurology. 2009;51(1):30-8.

[56] Militerni R, Bravaccio C, Falco C, Fico C, Palermo MT. Repetitive behaviors in autistic disorder. European Child & Adolescent Psychiatry. 2002;11(5):210-8.

[57] Bodfish JW, Symons FJ, Parker DE, Lewis MH. Varieties of Repetitive Behavior in Autism: Comparisons to Mental Retardation. Journal of Autism and Developmental Disorders. 2000;30(3):237-43.

[58] Van Hasselt VB, Hersen M, Egan BS, Mckelvey JL, Sisson LA. Increasing Social Interactions in Deaf-Blind Severely Handicapped Young Adults. Behavior Modification. 1989 April 1, 1989;13(2):257-72.

[59] Jan JE, Freeman RD, Scott EP. Visual impairment in children and adolescents. New York, NY: Grune & Stratton; 1977.

[60] Tröster H, Brambring M, Beelmann A. Prevalence and situational causes of stereotyped behaviors in blind infants and preschoolers. Journal of Abnormal Child Psychology. 1991;19(5):569-90.

[61] Tröster H, Brambring M, Beelmann A. The age dependence of stereotyped behaviours in blind infants and preschoolers. Child: Care, Health and Development. 1991;17(2):137-57.

[62] Murdoch H. Stereotyped Behaviours: How Should We Think About Them? British Journal of Special Education. 1997;24(2):71-5.

[63] Kraijer D, Bildt A. The PDD-MRS: An Instrument for Identification of Autism Spectrum Disorders in Persons with Mental Retardation. Journal of Autism and Developmental Disorders. 2005;35(4):499-513.

[64] Matson JL, Boisjoli JA. Autism spectrum disorders in adults with intellectual disability and comorbid psychopathology: Scale development and reliability of the ASD-CA. Research in Autism Spectrum Disorders. 2008;2(2):276-87.

[65] Roper L, Arnold P, Monteiro B. Co-Occurrence of Autism and Deafness. Autism. 2003 September 1, 2003;7(3):245-53.

[66] Mason J, Scior K. 'Diagnostic Overshadowing' Amongst Clinicians Working with People with Intellectual Disabilities in the UK. Journal of Applied Research in Intellectual Disabilities. 2004;17(2):85-90.

[67] Peters-Scheffer N, Didden R, Korzilius H, Sturmey P. A meta-analytic study on the effectiveness of comprehensive ABA-based early intervention programs for children with Autism Spectrum Disorders. Research in Autism Spectrum Disorders. 2011;5(1): 60-9.

[68] Peters-Scheffer N, Didden R, Green VA, Sigafoos J, Korzilius H, Pituch K, et al. The behavior flexibility rating scale-revised (BFRS-R): Factor analysis, internal consistency, inter-rater and intra-rater reliability, and convergent validity. Research in Developmental Disabilities. 2008;29(5):398-407.

Chapter 5

Clinical Implications of a Link Between Fetal Alcohol Spectrum Disorders (FASD) and Autism or Asperger's Disorder – A Neurodevelopmental Frame for Helping Understanding and Management

Kieran D. O'Malley

Additional information is available at the end of the chapter

1. Introduction

The teratogenic effect of alcohol was first observed by paediatrician Paul Lemoine in Nantes, France in 1968, when he linked facial dysmorphic and growth features with maternal use of alcohol (wine) in pregnancy. His initial series was 127 infants. Subsequently the syndrome Fetal Alcohol Syndrome was defined in 2 classic papers in 1973 by David smith and Ken Jones in Seattle. Their initial case series were 8 patients. The recognition that prenatal alcohol exposure did not just cause dysmorphic facial features and growth delay was made by Sterling Clarren in Seattle in 1978 with the introduction of the term Fetal Alcohol Effect (FAE) to describe children with alcohol exposure but no facial features. This descriptive clinical term was changed to Alcohol Related Neurodevelopmental Disorder (ARND) by the Institute of Medicine in 1996.

2. A conceptual understanding of the spectrum of effects of prenatal alcohol exposure

In the same vein as Autistic Spectrum Disorders, Fetal Alcohol Spectrum Disorders (FASD,) initially described by Streissguth & O'Malley in 2000 is an umbrella term to describe the continuum of complex neuropsychiatric, cognitive, behavioral, social, language, communication and other multi-sensory deficits. There are, however, two conditions within this spectrum which describe the range of conditions caused by prenatal alcohol exposure. They are Fetal

Alcohol Syndrome (FAS) a dysmorphic syndrome, and Alcohol Related Neurodevelopment Disorder (ARND) a non dysmorphic condition and by far the more common of the two conditions.

However within FASD there are physical sequellae aside from the facial dysmorphology, which are associated with all levels of prenatal alcohol exposure (Stratton et al 1996). These Alcohol Related Birth Defects (ARBD), as they are called, can occur as early as the first few weeks post conception.So, before most women know they are pregnant (Sulik, et al., 1983).

The central nervous system (CNS) and brain are the most sensitive and vulnerable structures to the effects of alcohol and can be affected by moderate to heavy alcohol use at any point in gestation. There is no safe amount of alcohol (threshold) during pregnancy and the Surgeon General of the United States currently recommends all childbearing age women to avoid alcohol if there is a potential for pregnancy (US Surgeon General, 2005).

Early, frequent, and/or binge exposures with moderate to high blood alcohol concentrations can lead to a range of reproductive outcomes including infertility, miscarriage (spontaneous fetal loss), still birth, sudden infant death syndrome, and a wide range of physical and neurodevelopmental (functional) birth defects. Varying degrees of Fetal Alcohol Syndrome (FAS) may be seen clinically at this range of exposure (Jones & Smith 1973, Streissguth et al 1987, 1991). Alcohol-Related Neurodevelopmental Disorder (ARND, Stratton et al., 1996) are the neurodevelopmental/functional birth defects that manifest in individuals with FAS, as well as those who do not meet full criteria for FAS but have documented evidence of prenatal alcohol exposure. ARND can be associated with inattention, poor decision making, impulsivity, processing and working memory issues, other areas of executive dysfunction, mood instability, social communication deficits, and difficulties understanding consequences of their actions. These deficits are best evaluated by a thorough neuropsychological exam, including the Vineland Adaptive behavioral scales, IQ testing, and assessment of executive functions, such as BRIEF., FASD includes two conditions FAS which is dysmorphic and ARND, which is non-dysmorphic (See Table 1.).

Both FAS, dysmorphic and ARND. non-dysmorphic conditions can be associated with physical sequellae resulting from alcohol exposure in pregnancy. The Institute of Medicine describes these physical manifestations collectively as Alcohol Related Birth Defects (ARBD), including abnormalities in the developing eye, ear, teeth, heart, kidney, and skeletal system (Stratton et al, 1996; O'Malley & Streissguth, 2000; Chudley et al, 2005; BMA, 2007). Like the typical FAS facial features, ARBD occur in the first 8 weeks of embryonic development (organogenesis). Many of these conditions may not be diagnosed or evident at the time of a patient's psychiatric evaluation (Iich 2005, Nowick Brown et al 2011).

The major difference between dysmorphic (i.e., FAS) and nondysmorphic (ARND) phenotypes is whether or not the collective cardinal (dysmorphic) facial features are present. The facial features correlate to heavy maternal blood alcohol concentration (e.g., the equivalent of 5 to 6 servings of alcohol) during the earliest points in gestation (late 3rd week to early 4th week of embryonic development) (Sulik, 1983). Both the facial features and ARBD are due to early embryonic changes, disruptions in cell migration, and cell death (apoptosis) due to the teratogenic effects of alcohol. Thus, the clinical relevance of both ARBD and the facial features in FAS is that of biomarkers for heavy binge exposure early in pregnancy – and sometimes, but not always, may predict a worse neurodevelopmental prognosis (Riley and McGee, 2005, Coles et al 2011). Since both FAS and ARND have neurodevelopmental (CNS) involvement, essentially ARND is FAS without the characteristic facial features. (Rich& O'Malley 2012).

A. Fetal Alcohol Syndrome (FAS), a specific dysmorphic phenotype, requires documentation of all of the following clinical features.

• may or may not have a clear history of documented maternal alcohol use in pregnancy;

• dysmorphic facial features based on racial norms (including all of the following: small palpebral fissures at or below 10th percentile, smooth philtrum, thin vermillion border) – this requires a clinical dysmorphologist with an understanding of FAS diagnosis;

• growth problems: confirmed prenatal or postnatal height or weight, or both, at or below the 10th percentile, documented at any one point in time (adjusted for age, sex, gestational age, and race or ethnicity).

• Central Nervous System (CNS) abnormalities:

I. Structural:

A. Head circumference (OFC) at or below the 10th percentile adjusted for age and sex.

B. Clinically significant brain abnormalities observable through imaging.

II. Neurological problems not due to a postnatal insult or fever, or other soft neurological signs outside normal limits.

III. Functional Performance substantially below that expected for an individual's age, schooling, or circumstances, as evidenced by:

A. Global cognitive or intellectual deficits representing multiple domains of deficit (or significant developmental delay in younger children) with performance below the 3rd percentile (2 standard deviations below the mean for standardized testing) or

B. Functional deficits below the 16th percentile (1 standard deviation below the mean for standardized testing) in at least three of the following domains:

1. cognitive or developmental deficits or discrepancies

2. executive functioning deficits

3. motor functioning delays

4. problems with attention or hyperactivity

5. social skills

6. other clinically relevant neurodevelopmental issues (i.e., sensory problems, pragmatic language problems, memory deficits, etc.)

B. Alcohol Related Neurodevelopmental Disorder (ARND) is a non-dysmorphic condition with the following features:

• must have a documented history of maternal alcohol use during pregnancy;

• none or not all pathognomonic dysmorphic facial features are present;
• no evidence of growth delay, low birth weight, decelerating weight over time, nor other height and weight issues;
• Central Nervous System (CNS) abnormalities:
I. Structural:
A. Head circumference (OFC) at or below the 10th percentile adjusted for age and sex.
B. Clinically significant brain abnormalities observable through imaging.
II. Neurological problems not due to a postnatal insult or fever, or other soft neurological signs outside normal limits.
III. Functional Performance substantially below that expected for an individual's age, schooling, or circumstances, as evidenced by:
A. Global cognitive or intellectual deficits representing multiple domains of deficit (or significant developmental delay in younger children) with performance below the 3rd percentile (2 standard deviations below the mean for standardized testing) or
B. Functional deficits below the 16th percentile (1 standard deviation below the mean for standardized testing) in at least three of the following domains:
1. cognitive or developmental deficits or discrepancies
2. executive functioning deficits
3. motor functioning delays
4. problems with attention or hyperactivity
5. social skills
6. other clinically relevant neurodevelopmental issues (i.e., sensory problems, pragmatic language problems, memory deficits, etc.)

(Jones & Smith 1973, 1975, Stratton et al 1996, Chudney et al 2005, BMA 2007, O'Malley 2008, Novick Brown et al 2011, O'Malley & Mukarjee 2010, CDC 2011,HHS)

Table 1. Characteristic Diagnostic Features of FAS (dysmorphic) and ARND (non dysmorphc)

Among both phenotypes, FAS is the less common condition, accounting for only 20-25% of the affected infants and children exposed to all levels of alcohol exposure. By comparison, non-dysmorphic ARND is the more common clinical presentation of affected infants and children, accounting for 75 to 80% of affected infants exposed to all levels of alcohol in pregnancy. While maternal alcohol use is the leading known preventable cause of mental retardation and birth defects, only 20-25% of patients with either dysmorphic FAS or nondysmorphic ARND have a total IQ below 70. In other words, 75 to 80% of patients with FASD are estimated to have a developmental disability or other CNS impairment (acquired brain injury) but are not mentally retarded (Streissguth et al., 1996; Mukarjee et al., 2006). Hence FASD (FAS and ARND) are NOT mental retardation conditions, but are complex neurodevelopmental disorders with initial developmental, cognitive, and neurobehavioral outcomes, and higher lifetime risk of psychiatric co-morbidities and substance use disorders.

The dysmorphic facial appearance of an individual is much less an impact than the complex behaviors, psychopathology and developmental disability caused by alcohol's neurotoxicity. Thus, an individual's level of functioning is affected more by behavioral functioning, intellect, cognitive and communication abilities, executive functioning, temperament, social related-ness, emotional regulation, and performance than what his or her face looks like. FAS, the dysmorphic presentation of ARND, is in fact a protective factor for what Ann Streissguth called secondary disabilities of FASD (Streissguth et al 1996).

Neuroimaging studies suggest that alcohol exposure may be specific rather than global in its teratogenicity, including specific vulnerability in the cerebellum, basal ganglia, and corpus callosum. As well, studies have shown deficits in cognitive functions such as learning and memory, visual-spatial functioning, executive functioning, attention, sequencing, processing and motor control. (Mattson et al 2011) These "functional birth defects" are evidenced by impairment in the brain and central nervous system. Riley and colleagues have shown that functional birth defects are present in children with moderate to heavy prenatal alcohol exposure, even in absence of characteristic (dysmorphic) facial features (Bookstein et al 2001, Riley and McGee, 2005, Coles et al 2011).

It is a critical issue in clinical diagnosis of FASD to understand that the severity of the acquired brain injury is not always correlated with the presence of facial dysmorphology (and FAS facial features commonly change significantly in adolescence and adulthood). Therefore facial features are minimally useful to assess and treat neurocognitive and neurobehavioral deficits associated with prenatal alcohol exposure. (Streissguth, et al., 1991; Steinhausen, et al., 1993, Nowick Brown et al 2011, Kodituwakku et al 2011, O'Malley 2011, Rich & O'Malley 2012).

The first 30 to 40 years of research in FASD has been driven by animal teratology and the pursuit of minute changes in facial dysmorphology as biological markers for the level of prenatal alcohol exposure. Nevertheless, it is becoming quite clear that it is the central nervous system brain dysfunction that is the kernel of the problem and the guide to diagnostic understanding and management. It is not the face that tells the clinician about the underlying brain dysfunction but the complex mixture of developmental disability and psychiatric disorder. FASD, whether dysmorphic FAS or non dysmorphic ARND are developmental psychiatric disorders which, as Susan Rich and Kieran O'Malley describe in their 2012 paper. These conditions can present a neurodevelopmental mixture of mood dysregulation and autonomic arousal with language and social skills deficits, cognitive and executive decision making dysfunctions and multisensory functional and perceptual deficits

2.1. The link between FASD and autism or Asperger's disorder

As far back as 1990, child neuropsychologist Jo Nanson in Saskatoon, Canada, described 6 cases of FAS with autism. As well, the interest in prenatal risk factors contributing to autism has been pursued by a number of authors and this potential aetiological link was published in 1991 by International autism researcher Cathy Lord and colleagues. More recently, since

2009-2010, adult psychiatrist in London, Raja Mukarjee, has painstakingly clinically analysed the clinical presentation of Autistic Spectrum Disorder in patients with FASD.

In the international paediatric and child psychiatric field the last 5 years have brought a wealth of clinical case descriptions and case studies indicating the presence of ADHD co-morbidly with PDD or Autistic Spectrum Disorder. Clinicians and researchers such as Professor Jeremy Turk in the UK have commented on as much as a 25-30% co-morbid link between ADHD and PDD/ASD. Furthermore the complexity of diagnostic issues within FASD have been recently illustrated in a 2011 on line book chapter by Natalie Novick Brown, Kieran O'Malley and Ann Streissguth in which the developmental psychiatric presentations of FASD were shown to include sometimes unrecognized Autistic Spectrum Disorder or Asperger's Disorder.

2.2. Aetiological theories postulated for this link

It is important to place the possible link between prenatal alcohol exposure and Autism spectrum disorder or Asperger's Disorder in a historical context. Environmental agents, diseases and postnatal interventions have had, it is fair to say, a rather mixed and controversial past, as recently pointed out by Cathy Lord, So Hyun K im and Adriana Dimartino in 2011.

Although as far back as 1971 American child psychiatrist Stella Chess's case review of rubella and thalidomide cases implicated these prenatal infectious and medication exposures as aetiological, the series were small. European researchers Gilberg and Gilberg in 1983 have more rigorously identified a cluster of adverse prenatal complications which may contribute to a clinical presentation of Autism Spectrum disorder in early childhood.

However the most studied, but as well the most problematic, was the potential association between MMR vaccine and Autism Spectrum Disorder. It is not the remit of the chapter to completely review this, ultimately, false trail. Nevertheless it offers a salutary lesson in the emotional reactions that possible environmental agents or interventions can elicit to the public at large, but also the medical profession.

Alcohol has been in society for ever and the acknowledgement of prenatal alcohol and its tertatogenic effect is still relatively a new phenomenon. So it is prudent to not 'scaremonger', but scientifically and clinically carefully piece out the veracity of this possible link.

The science of alcohol teratology continues to advance in leaps and bounds and one of the core findings has been the effect of prenatal alcohol on the dynamic balance of the developing neurotransmitters. In parallel with the more focused autism research on the role of serotoninergic neurotransmitters has been the identified effect of alcohol on the embryological serotoninergic neurotransmitter system. This research branches into the study of the serotonin transporter gene, by groups such as Bonnin et al in 2011, but again parallel work on epigenetics in alcohol has begun to unravel probable trans-generational shifts in genetic transcription through effects on DNA methylation (Haycock 2009).

Another strand of research in alcohol teratogenesis has been identifying brain areas a more sensitive to alcohol damage. Areas such as the corpus callosum, hippocampus, prefrontal cortex, temporal lobe collectively and individually contribute to a clinical presentation of social disconnectedness, lack of social cognition and awareness, impulsivity, and inability to understand another person's cognitions or feelings (alexithymia). (Bookstein et al 2001).

The underlying organic brain dysfunction at a cellular, neurotransmitter and structural level related to prenatal alcohol exposure sometimes shares significant congruence with ongoing neuroscience research in Autism Spectrum Disorder and Asperger's Disorder, and awaits collaborative work between the two academic fields.

There is also accumulating research which highlights the biological roots of fundamental functional problems in FASD which relate to sustained impact on working memory, (Congdon et al 2012)

2.3. Neuropsychological framework of understanding ASD and Aspergers and its relationship to patients with FASD

1. The psychological deficit in the child must be present before the onset of the disorder and so very early in development.

2. Be pervasive among individuals with the disorder.

3. Be specific to autism

4. Different psychological theories

   a. theory of mind theory

   b. the executive theory

   c. the praxis/imitation theory

   d. the emotion theory

   e. the emphathizing-systematizing or ' extreme male brain' theory (Hobson 1989, Russell 1997, Baren Cohen et al 2000, Pennington 2009)

2.4. Clinical presentations of Aspergers disorder or autism spectrum disorder with FASD

This is the arena where the divergence between the classic presentations of Autism Spectrum Disorder and Aspergers Disorder are seen, and offer a way to untangle the different aetiological routes to these syndromes.

FASD begin at birth and can be seen in infancy. The Mental Health Classification system, Zero to three (DC 0-3R, 2005) has a diagnostic category of Regulatory Disorders which aptly describes the immediate clinical presentations of Dysmorphic FAS or non dysmorphic ARND. It is the category of Regulatory Disorder, underresponsive type which is the harbinger of autism Spectrum Disorder or Aspergers Disorder diagnoses in early child hood.So the classic time presentation of Autism Spectrum Disorder or Aspergers Disorder is different in the FASD population.

The stereotypic movements, flapping, posturing are less commonly part of the FASD presentation. However they present more commonly a Developmental Co-ordination Disorder which is diagnosed often Dyspraxia in countries such as Ireland.

The essence of the overlapping clinical presentations comes in the expressive and receptive language area. The qualitative impairments in social awareness, social cognition, social communication are not uncommonly very hard to differentiate whether using clinical assessment by an experienced child psychiatrist or psychologist or using standardized instruments such as ADOS among others. In many countries the ambivalence to accept the true prevalence of FASD(! in 100 live births) leads school systems and physicians to 'hide' many FASD patients under a Autism Spectrum Disorder or Asperger's Disorder diagnosis because of the expediency of receiving school learning disability services. This is slowly changing, pioneered in countries such as Canada and the USA. Now the UK are acknowledging that FASD are the current biggest challenge for teaching as these pupils display complex learning disabilities with co –morbid psychiatric disorders for which there is no regular curriculum (Professor Barry Carpenter UK, 2012).

This chapter will include psychiatric clinical analysis of patients with FASD who present autism spectrum Disorder or Aspergers Disorder features. with formal cognitive testing done and not uncommonly differing autism assessments which have proved equivocal. The co-morbid ADHD is a more frequent issue in the FASD population and this has critical importance in both understanding and management. For example a successful medication treatment of pervasive distractibility visual and auditory can have a positive effect on the child's social functioning as he/she can now attend sufficiently to read faces and verbal and non verbal cues.

Medication is a change in the FASD patients who present with Autism spectrum disorder or Aspergers Disorder features. The more commonly accepted efficacy of SSRI does not necessarily hold true for FASD children or adolescents with and can lead to unmasking a bipolar diathesis, or in older patients contributing to Extra pyramidal symptoms.. This is especially a problem in Ireland which has a high prevalence of Affective Disorder which is quite common in the mothers who drink alcohol during pregnancy and so this genetic vulnerability can be brought forth by too aggressive use of SSRI for that autism or Aspergers Disorder. As well the psychostimulants can lead to an over focus in the FASD/ ASD group with increased perseveration which can become a source of severe rage if challenged. As well the psychostimulants are more likely to run the risk of bringing a schizoid change in the patient. Atypical agents such as risperidone with its differential effect on 5HT receptor can also prove problematic in management of Autism or Aspergers with a prenatal alcohol exposure history. In this case the longer and prolonged use of the medicine can make the clinical situation worse by unmasking an affective instability. (Rich & O'Malley 2012)

Seizure disorders can be related to prenatal alcohol exposure and the effect of alcohol on the GABA ergic system is one hypothesis. (Daniel Bonthius et al 1992, O'Malley and Barr 1998).unexplained explosive episodes, rage attacks in FASD patients with autism Spectrum disorder or Aspergers Disorder may have origins in seizure disorders which are not related to the lower level of cognitive functioning or IQ as is the accepted rule.

Little comment is made on the family stress in this complex mix population but a family centred therapeutic approach is the kernel of management and Identity issues have a completely different resonance in an adolescent who is bright, has ARND, Aspergers disorder and is trying to cope with the early loss of a birth mother to cirrhosis of the liver at 36 when her/she is aware that the ARND has its roots in the birth mothers drinking during pregnancy. In Ireland the 3/4 generations of families with FASD creates a transgenerational challenge to unraveling disorganized parenting from disconnected parenting due to fundamental social communication disorders. (Cummings et al 2000)

Recent international guidelines have included FASD among the environmentally-induced neurodevelopmental disorders. (Sage Handbook of Developmental Disorders, 2011) Such a neurodevelopmental diagnostic framework for children and adolescents with FASD improves outcome and prognosis in many cases, notably for those with persistent aggressive and antisocial behaviors. Neither the dysmorphic, Fetal Alcohol Syndrome (FAS) nor the non-dysmorphic,Alcohol Related Neurodevelopmental Disorder (ARND) condition is currently diagnosable as an Axis I disorder.

Therefore Susan Rich and Kieran O'Malley, 2012, have recently proposed an alternative psychiatric formulation based on a neurodevelopmental model. This was suggested in order to improve clinical understanding and treatment of these complex developmental psychiatric patients. Such a paradigm shift would better identify the large numbers of children who fall through the cracks in diagnostic coding, becoming stuck in a revolving door through psychiatric hospitals and institutions. (Brown et al 2011).

These complex cognitive and psychiatric deficits often predispose affected individuals to a high degree of sensitivity to medications, increased risk of overmedication, treatment with medication combinations, susceptibility to changes in dosing regimens, and paradoxical responses to certain drugs.

Increasing clinical experience in using a neurodevelopmental formulation (compared to the traditional multi-axial system) to guide the measured, educated use of psychotropics for treatment of FASD can facilitate dramatic improvements in functioning of this challenging population.

Early and/or multidisciplinary intervention and treatment can prevent or minimize disruptive and risky behaviors, reduce academic failure, improve placement outcomes and reduce chronic involvement in the legal and probation system. (O'Malley 2011b, Rich & O'Malley 2012)

3. The domains of alcohol-related neurodevelopmental disorder

Although nearly every type of Axis I and II disorder in both DSM IV –TR and ICD 10 Classifications, as well as most disorders from the 0-3 coding manual can be expressed by individuals with effects of prenatal alcohol exposure, there have been efforts to better characterize the common clinical features associated with ARND. While neurodevelopmental deficits may exist in a range of severity, all cases of individuals with FAS have some degree of ARND. The following neurodevelopmental domains have been found to be disrupted in clinical psychiatric cases of both FAS and ARND (Figure 1). As indicated in the diagram, prenatal alcohol exposure can lead to mood dysregulation and autonomic arousal, cognitive and executive dysfunctions, language and social skills deficits, and multi-sensory functional and perceptual deficits. Some individuals can have one or more domains of impairment, as indicated by the overlapping areas in the Venn diagram. (Rich et al 2009, Solomon et al 2009, Rich & O'Malley 2012)

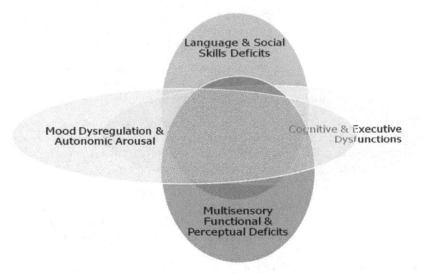

Figure 1. Mood dysregulation and/or Autonomic Arousal:

It is slowly being recognized that the autonomic or involuntary (parasympathetic and sympathetic) nervous system is affected by prenatal alcohol exposure, Animal research indicated this many years ago but human studies are beginning to unravel its effect from the infancy, early child hood and through to adolescence. Regulatory Disorders are prime clinical examples of this effect of prenatal alcohol exposure. The classic dichotomy in temperament is seen in the predisposition for a hyporesponsive infant or child, shy, inhibited, cautious and, anxious or hyperreponsive, a dis-inhibited, impulsive, intense infant or child. the effect of alcohol on the CNS produces a highly mood dysregulated child, having random or easily provoked episodes of frustration, irritability, aggression, and anger. Infants and toddlers with FASD can present with Regulatory Disorder Type I, II, or III (DC Zero to Three, 2005). The type of mood dysregulation may be related to "brain irritability" as epileptiform activity and spike and wave forms can be seen in sleep deprived or 24-hour EEGs for some individuals. This phenomenon is akin to a faulty thermostat which instead of controlling temperature controls emotional and arousal regulation. Thus the patient is unable to adjust their emotional or arousal state appropriately in response to sometimes minor challenges i.e. failure of examination, break up from boyfriend. This can lead to emotional incontinence with uncontrollable crying or laughing, or maybe intermittent unpredictable explosive episodes.

These developmental psychiatric disorders presenting from infancy reflect the impact of prenatal alcohol on the developing neurotransmitter system. This teratogenic effect on the serotonin, GABA ergic Glutaminergic and other neurotransmitter systems can lead to anxiety disorders, mood disorders (such as depression), aggression, and possibly later substance abuse. As infants and toddlers, they are often temperamentally difficult to settle and do not seem to enjoy/bond with their parents, birth, foster or adoptive These infants may have pervasive sleep problems (with disruptions in the sleep/wake cycle, initial insomnia and decreased non REM sleep).As well they can display a whole range of regulatory problems in hyper or hyposensivity to auditory, visual,, olfactory, gustatory or tactile stimuli.

As young children, the sensory integration issues involving sensitivity to sounds, environmental noise, lights, fans, easily irritated by voices, loud music, smells, tastes, even touch continue, and are often misunderstood as deliberate defiance.

This is commonly a clinical arena in which so called 'autistic 'features are noticed. In other words, the young child with ARND may either seek out tactile stimulation (touch and/or movement) or may, alternatively, be sensitive to touch and/or easily over-aroused by vigorous proprioceptive stimuli (e.g., movement on swings, roller coasters, etc.).

Generally, transition periods are a challenge, not unlike autistic children. These children require intensive one-on-one adult attention being unable to self-soothe easily, and having difficulty in free /creative play. However, self regulation techniques can be taught and guide play therapy has a role in integration of the child's exploration of self expression.

3.1. Cognitive and executive dysfunction

Brain structural, neurophysiological or neurotransmitter abnormalities belie the cognitive deficits in ARND. These include: working memory deficits, difficulty with executive functioning (organization, concentration, auditory processing, processing speed, problem solving, attention and impulse control.); deficits in IQ compared with their biological parents; mathematics disorders, reading disorders (e.g., dyslexia), spelling issues, and other learning disabilities with or without mental retardation due to a hypoaroused, misconnected, or disconnected prefrontal cortex, individuals with ARND may have a variety of deficits in cognitive areas,. A variety of developmental disabilities (speech/language issues, visual integration, gross and/or fine motor skills deficits (i.e., poor handwriting), spasticity, hyperflexibility, etc.) can also be seen in many individuals with ARND.

Disruptions in cognitive functioning often lead to a failure to understand consequences, poor judgment, and limited insight into the origins or the impact of one's behaviors. This subsequently leads to significant and debilitating deficits in basic day to day functional abilities. The child with ARND therefore, rather than thinking through actions, acts impulsively often in a naïve/ primitive manner (as though driven by basic instinct rather than measured intellect).

Self care is another area of concern. able to care for oneself (e.g., hygiene, meal preparation, scheduling appointments), manage a household (take on responsibilities for chores, balance a checkbook, etc.) and perform other activities of daily living may be limited depending on the extent of a person's ARND.

Time, homework and money management difficulties lead to multitudes of practical daily living problems. Children with ARND are seen as willful, lazy and showing clear oppositional defiant features. The level of IQ does not offer a guide to these cognitive issues and often can suggest a greater capability than is possible. Children with ARND not uncommonly present a mixture of autistic features with ADHD and so are doubly challenged. Medication can have a vital role in this group as they are misunderstood as having faulty 'theory of mind' deficits, whereas their distractibility and lack of focus makes them unable to fully participate in social situation.

It is more common sense in the later grades/years in school to guide the student towards a vocational training certificate rather than a diploma/ A level, Leaving Certificate track and to master the basic life skills to be productive, employed in a semi-skilled trade (e.g., construction worker, brick mason, landscape worker, plumber's assistant, etc.). However, for many individuals with a higher degree of functioning and with appropriate academic/examination support it may not be unreasonable to expect completion of secondary/ high school and even the entering of a two or four year college or university programme. This is especially true for FAS or ARND patients with an autistic profile and average or above average intellectual functioning.

On the other hand, more cognitively impaired patients with FAS or ARND may have frequent rudimentary behaviors (skin picking, pica, compulsive self harm or inappropriate/self-stimulating sexual behaviors). These can be a primitive expression of emotional distress, not unlike non verbal autistic children. The central alexithymia, (inability to understand others feelings or have words for one's own feelings) irrespective of IQ level is a fundamental clinical construct in FASD.(Greene et al 1991)

3.2. Language and social skills deficits

The traditional view of language deficits come from the wealth of studies in expressive/ articulation problems and the more complicated so called 'receptive' language problems where the person has fundamental problems in the processing of language. this latter deficits was described by wernicke as long ago as 1874 in his classic treatise on sensory aphasia. It is in this area that patients withFASD truly show their 'autistic type clinical features. misuse of language integral to social cognition and communication are quite common problems in adolescents or young adults with ARND. It is important to understand that prenatal alcohol-induced organic brain damage underpins the language deficits. At times, these patients are misdiagnosed with Autistic Spectrum Disorder or Asperger's Disorder. The term "social language disorder" better fits this population. This does not preclude the fact that medication may engender a positive effect on language functioning, and specifically social communication. Individuals with ARND suffer from indiscriminate or immature behaviors (e.g., telling inappropriate jokes in the classroom or workplace, blurting out what they think of a person even if it is quite insulting /silly or negative). These behavior problems range from silly or irritating socially inappropriate behaviors to overtly aggressive and sometimes risky behaviors. Severe social functioning problems may result in lack of long term friendships, being labeled by peers as "weird" or "odd," and/or appearing withdrawn, socially-isolated, and avoidant. At times, ARND may lead to socially indiscriminate behaviors (i.e., individuals engaging in early or promiscuous sexual activity, gang membership, and peer pressure).

The clinical understanding of the effect of pseudo word decoding and alexithymia in management and understanding is critical to the psychiatrist, psychologist and educator. These children and adolescents can be seen in an 'autistic' or 'defiant' light but have specific decoding struggles which effect their receptive).

Case Examples: Two female adolescents with ARND were diagnosed with Autism and Atypical Autism respectively after fulfilling the ADOS criteria. However both had clear documented history of prenatal alcohol exposure. One normal I.Q. I4 year old girl with Atypical Autism had a clinical presentation of ASD and ADD and deteriorated with psychostimulant medication which markedly increased her perseveration. She responded to low dose liquid fluoxetine, and as her attention problems, especially visual, ameliorated, so her 'autistic' features deceased. The other girl 15 years old, with moderate intellectual functioning, had very debilitating social anxiety triggered by oversensitivity to facial cues. She eventually settled for a while with a GABA ergic agent.(Lyrica, pregabulin), but now needs a specialized therapeutic community placement. She had a history of many unexplained physical problems which were Alcohol Related Birth Defects.

3.3. Multi-sensory functional and perceptual deficits

Sensory integration issues, including hypo or hypersensitivities to noise, touch, proprioceptive stimuli, smells, tastes, and light may all be seen in children prenatally exposed to alcohol. This may lead to infants and toddlers seeming to be easily agitated, over-stimulated, and over-aroused. Adolescents and adults may cope by avoiding or over-reacting in situations or environments which provoke their sensitivities. Adolescents or adults who misread or misunderstand social cues may result in paranoid behaviors, such as over-reactions to the tone of someone's voice or an otherwise harmless look in their direction.

Prenatal alcohol exposure can have very disabling outcomes for alcohol-exposed children and their families due to the interaction between psychosocial risk factors (Mukarjee et al, 2006), cognitive deficits, and neuropsychiatric sequelae (O'Malley 2011b). In addition to a higher prevalence of chronic exposure to domestic violence, neglect, child abuse, adjudicated youth have higher rates of psychiatric illness, learning disabilities, and academic failure.

The sensory functional and perceptual deficits are commonly' hidden' and included in a generic autistic diagnosis frame. However they are fundamental to understanding the acquired brain damage caused by alcohol, which pervades brain structures, neurotransmitters and electrophysiology (Hagerman 1999, O'Malley 2008, O'Malley & Mukarjee 2010).

Case example: A 21 year old previously adopted male Caucasian patient presented with a long history of autism and psychotic features. He had been hospitalized a number of times and had need restraint because of his reactivity to the environment. He had not responded to high doses of SSRIs (which produced increased suicidality thoughts), and atypical, especially risperidone which made him more affectively unmanageable. When he was assessed in the community his clear history of sensory reactivity to tactile, olfactory, gustatory, visual and auditory stimuli was unraveled as was his history of significant prenatal alcohol exposure. Which had been ignored in previous assessments. A combined multi-modal approach addressing his sensory reactivity combined with low dose buspirione was much more effective and he did not need psychiatric hospitalization. As well he did not present any facial features as adult or as a young child. He had been labeled as having unusual paranoid features but these were really his correct sensitivity to what he perceived as a hostile challenging environment. His adoptive parents recounted many stories of his oversensitivity to noise, light,fabrics food when he was growing op and just saw him as 'over fussy'.

4. A neurodevelopmenatal approach to management

4.1. General diagnostic problems

Although psychiatrists and mental health professionals treat patients with FASD, there is presently no consistent way within DSM-IV TR to code for either the dysmorphic phenotype (Fetal Alcohol Syndrome, FAS) or the non-dysmorphic condition (Alcohol-related Neurode-velopmental Disorder, ARND). Therefore, treatment of affected individuals is inadequate due to lack of diagnostic clarity, and lack of scientifically tested or accepted psychiatric treatment protocols. FAS, the leading non-hereditary cause of mental retardation and preventable birth defects, is buried in Appendix G of the DSM-IV TR as a congenital malformation (760.71) and the ICD-10 includes Fetus and newborn affected by maternal use of alcohol (P04.3) but excludes FAS (Q86.0) (DSM IV-TR, 2000). (Nowick Brown et al 2011, O'Malley 2011b, Rich & O'Malley 2012).

At the current time because there is no appropriate DSM-IV TR or ICD 10 diagnostic frame-work, most psychiatrists and mental health professionals attempt to apply inadequate Axis I diagnoses which are often poorly suited to the clinical understanding of this population. This results in individuals being given a laundry list of psychiatric diagnoses, from ADHD, autism, pervasive developmental disorder and bipolar disorder, to conduct disorder, reactive attach-ment disorder, personality disorders, and oppositional defiant disorder.

In a large study of secondary disabilities in 415 persons with ARND [FAS or Fetal Alcohol Effect (FAE)], a majority (94%) had a history of co-occurring mental health problems. Among both adults and children, attention deficits were the most frequently reported problems (61%) reported whereas in adults alone, depression was most frequently reported (52%) (Stratton et al., 1996). A smaller study has shown that the proportion of subjects with a history of psychi-atric disorders (74%) was greater than expected from the general population, including alcohol or drug abuse (60%), major depressive disorder (44%), avoidant personality disorder (29%). Researchers have shown a link between ADHD symptoms and FASD over the past several years, indicating an acquired (non-genetic) etiology for a subtype of children with ADHD.

Infants and toddlers with FASD can present with Regulatory Disorder Type I, II, or III (DC Zero to 3, 2005). Autistic behaviors have been noted in both younger children as well as school age children prenatally exposed to alcohol (Streissguth et al, 1996; Streissguth & O'Malley, 2000, Mukarjee et al 2012).

You could build a case that nearly all disorders developing during childhood listed in the DSM IV-TR may be induced by exposure to alcohol in utero. Co-morbidities of FASD include other behavioral, mood, anxiety, and conduct problems. The link between ADHD and FASD is finding more universal acceptance and the link between autism and Aspergers disorder and FASD will not be far behind. (O'Malley 2011a).The lifetime prevalence of mental health or psychiatric disorders in individuals with FASD is as high as 90% (Streissguth et al 1996, HHS, 2000), highlighting the importance of correct diagnosis and clinical management. Accurate, informed diagnosis is critical in psychiatry to avoid over-medication or inappropriate treatment, leading to worsening of symptoms and poor outcomes.

The current standard of care or "treatment as usual" for individuals with FASD is inadequate due to lack of diagnostic clarity, lack of accepted psychiatric treatment protocols, and further complicated by the presence of Alcohol Related Birth Defects (ARBD) which are multisystem organ involvement (i.e., seizure disorders; renal, eye, cardiac, g.i. problems and skeletal).

Early accurate diagnosis and intervention may be effective in preventing the development of secondary disabilities (i.e., academic or school failure, conduct disorders and antisocial behaviours leading to legal problems, sexually inappropriate behaviours, lack of steady employment and housing).

4.2. The utilization of a neurodevelopmental formulation

The utilization of a neurodevelopmental formulation can guide the development of effective multiisystem and multimodal intervention strategies, including appropriate psychopharmacologic management (O'Malley 2008).

1. Thus, shifting diagnostic paradigms in children with prenatal alcohol exposure to the dysmorphic (FAS) and non-dysmorphic (ARND) phenotypic expression of in utero alcohol exposure would allow psychiatrists, pediatricians, and other medical professionals to have a richer, clearer and more holistic interpretation and understanding of the wide range of neurocognitive, neurobehavioral, and neuropsychiatric disorders affecting the individual rather than simply the degree of facial dysmorphology.

2. The social or environmental context includes childhood exposure to domestic or community violence, child abuse/neglect, early institutionalization, community violence, and other early life events that may contribute to development of reactive attachment disorder (RAD), post traumatic stress disorder (PTSD), developmental trauma disorder and other psychiatric (Axis I and II) co-morbidities.

The interaction of the childhood experience on the expressed FASD phenotype cannot be overlooked. Therefore, the neurodevelopmental biological vulnerability profile of FASD during infancy, toddlerhood, childhood, and adolescence predisposes an individual to adverse psychological outcomes resulting from early institutionalization, parental loss, physical/emotional/sexual abuse, neglect, and other forms of trauma(Cummings et al 2000,Elias et al 2011, Rich & O'Malley 2012).

3. 3.The implications of FASD on development, behavior, academic and adaptive functioning over the life span can be best understood in the context of the interaction of social and familial factors with an individual's neurodevelopmental deficits. Early institutionalization, neglect, abuse, and family violence may engender different nosological (diagnostic) presentations in this patient population, depending on the quality and degree of underlying neurodevelopmental impairment. So co-occurring diagnosis of Reactive Attachment Disorder or Post Traumatic Stress Disorder, Developmental Trauma Disorder are quite appropriate and herald the psychiatric and care complexities of the patient. It is therefore of vital importance that care must be taken to tease out symptoms based on acquired developmental versus social history in order to develop a holistic, appropriate understanding of the interplay between brain-based and environmental (post-natal) origins of psychopathology.

4. Deficits in emotional regulation and mood, implicit ability to comprehend the nuances of social situations, auditory or visual information processing, functional working memory, and/or other executive functions put individuals at risk for further psychopathology in the face of environmental stressors. These neurodevelopmental (CNS) and psychiatric sequellae persist through the life course and may progress to worsening conditions with devastating outcomes and poor prognosis (Streissguth and O'Malley, 2000, Rich & O'Malley 2012).

A neurodevelopmental formulation provides the best option for clinical understanding of these types of FASD complex cases, but especially if autistic features are the presentation, and the patient has borderline or low intellectual function or a marked split (12-15 points) between verbal and performance I.Q. (O'Malley 2008, Chapter 1)

4.3.The practical utility of a neurodevelopmental approach

The challenges in the treatment of FASD currently relate to their clinical presentations having an array of apparent psychiatric co-morbidity, and a general lack of diagnostic clarity. In practice in both North America and Ireland/ UK clinicians who recognize the clinical significance of FAS or ARND, are given a number of psychiatric diagnoses (ADHD, Autism, Aspergers disorder, intermittent explosive disorder, conduct disorder, mood disorder, etc.). It is becoming increasingly evident that early onset dysregulation, social communication and forensic issues are presenting complex mixtures of biological and environmental vulnerabilities which display developmentally changing clinical presentations. The autistic presentation coupled with ADHD symptoms and intermittent unexplained explosive episodes is particularly perplexing and hard to manage. Thus, given that both conditions are common presentations of FAS and ARND (Fitzgerald M, 2010). Clinicians using a neurodevelopmental approach will have more success in understanding and treatment of FASD.

Multi-modal treatment can improve the developmental, social, academic, and mental health trajectory of these children (O'Malley 2008, Nowick Brown et al 2011). Brain organization and function is affected in many individuals with FASD/ARND and can be enhanced by appropriate multi-modal treatment strategies.

As with Autistic Spectrum Disorders, FASD diagnosis and treatment involves early intervention with a multimodal team approach (genetics, developmental pediatrics, psychologists, psychiatrists, PT/OT, speech, special education) (O'Malley 2008, 2011b, Kodituwakku et al 2011).

A capacity for consequential thinking is a key requirement for "decisional capacity." This is an expectation for adolescents or young adults in the school, work legal system, who have been involved in antisocial and/or violent acts. Unfortunately, due to the neurocognitive deficits associated with ARND, these individuals are often mentally and emotionally disconnected from the consequences of their actions, misread social cues, are easily frustrated and provoked, and are unable to navigate logical decision making. So called 'high functioning 'autistic patients fit this neurocognitive profile and have the added challenge of unexpected response to medication because of unrecognized brain damage (Coles et al 2009, Kodituwakku et al 2011, Hosenbucus et al 2012).

4.4. The specific use of medication in FASD with or without autistic features

Clinical experience has shown that proper medication combined with comprehensive, early intervention services will improve their neurodevelopmental and psychiatric outcomes. To that end, psychotropic medication can be viewed as an integral part of multi-modal management program for dysmorphic and non-dysmorphic ARND (FAS Diagnosis, 2005; Byrne 2008, Coles 2009; Novick Brown, et al., 2011).

4.4.1. Off — Label or off license use of psychopharmaceuticals in patients with FASD

No National Institute of Mental Health (NIMH), NICE (UK), or industry-sponsored studies exist on the safety and efficacy of medication in children, adolescents, or adults with FASD, so this continues to be a barrier to measured and safe treatment for all individuals.

There is literature on the pharmacological management of ADHD, Autism, Fragile X, aggression and addictive disorders (Hagerman 1999, Lee et al 2001, Glancy et al 2002 a, b, Vocci et al 2005, Turk 2012), which is often mis-extrapolated to apply to individuals with FASD. Since there is no definitive diagnosis in the current DSM-IV TR for FASD outside of 760.71 (which is embedded in the ICD-9 codes in the Appendices under both "FAS" and "toxic exposure to alcohol in utero"), no impetus exists for large scale clinical trials in psychiatric and mental health research. Such controlled clinical studies are needed to determine "best practices," or even smaller studies to determine safety and efficacy, or to gain FDA or NICE guideline approval for use of the medications in this unique neurodevelopmental psychiatric patient population (Turk 2009). Presently, there currently are no FDA, AACAP, APA guidelines for medication usage in adolescents or young adults with FASD who present with neuropsychiatric disorders. Therefore, all medications are used "off label" or 'off license' in this population.

4.4.2. Caution in use of medication in ARND

While research is scarce in patients with FASD, this population may be even more vulnerable than those with brain injury sustained in the postnatal period, childhood, adolescence, or adulthood. Individuals with FASD, whether FAS or ARND, have had fetal whole-body exposure during prenatal development, leading to the potential for unrecognized Alcohol Related Birth Defects (ARBD) in a number of organ systems (kidney, heart, liver/g.i. system, eye, immune system, neurological) (Stratton et al 1996). These underlying problems with physical organs and structures may lead to unanticipated side effects to even low doses of medication.

For example

i.   cardiac problems such as conduction anomalies, structural defects, and pathologic murmurs may be linked with adverse events with stimulant medications.

ii.   Overt seizure disorders and irritability of the brain (associated with random and triggered electrical discharges) may be present due to neuro-anatomical changes in the ARND brain. Therefore, safety issues related to decreased seizure threshold for certain medications should be considered prior to treatment of this population. (O'Malley & Barr 1998, Hagerman 1999,Bonthius et al 2001

iii.   Other medical complications associated with alcohol-related birth defects (ARBD) need to be considered prior to beginning medication.

iv.   Therefore, caution in use of medications should be given due to the unique vulnerability of these patients for severe and catastrophic side effects of certain medications due to:

   • differential or paradoxical medication response ;

   • prenatal alcohol-induced neurochemical or structural CNS changes (i.e., acquired brain injury);

   • complications related to multisystem organ involvement (absorption, metabolic or elimination problems related to kidney, gastro-intestinal or liver problems related to ARBD);

   • an increased incidence of seizure disorders in this population (i.e., lower seizure thresh hold);

   • overall greater risk of side effects from multiple drug combinations, higher doses of medications, and sensitivity to psychopharmaceuticals.

4.4.3. Psychopharmacological targeting of neurodevelopmental deficits to improve current function and general prognosis

It is well recognized that patients with acquired brain injury respond differently to medications than individuals with no brain injury.

International clinical experience with this population indicates that individuals with alcohol-induced brain damage (FAS and ARND) often respond to medications similarly to those with other types of acquired or traumatic brain injury.

A prudent therapeutic approach in this group of patients is to streamline the numbers of medications the person is taking in order to reduce drug-drug interactions and prevent complications from over-medication (Stratton et al, 1996; O'Malley & Storoz 2003; Byrne 2008; O'Malley 2008).

Medications need to be started at low doses and increased slowly – with the goal of maximizing efficacy and minimizing side effects to the sensitive/vulnerable central nervous system. This can be achieved more often than not by simplifying the medication regimen, reducing the drug-drug interactions, and providing targeted therapy combined with medication management.

Psychotropic agents do improve brain organization and function (i.e., "neuron glue") and y can facilitate cognitive processes by dampening the spontaneous or random firing of mislaid pathways in the brain. As well, psychotropic medications may improve mood, behavior, and performance in individuals with FASD by altering the physiology of the "injured brain" structure and function. Among these medications are the atypical antipsychotics, such as risperdal, ziprazidone, aripiprizole, and olanzapine. Uses of lamotrigine, carbamazepine, valproic acid, lyrica, frisium have also been anecdotally helpful in patients with generalised anxiety, aggressively, impulsivity, and mood dysregulation. We believe that correctly chosen, appropriately managed medications can have a positive effect on cognitive functioning and decision making. (Hosenbus et al 2012, O'Malley 2010, Turk 2012).

4.4.4. General principles regarding medication usage in FASD

The principles guiding use of medications in the organically compromised brain (targeted medications, lower doses, and gradual increases in dosing) combined with psychotherapy and comprehensive community supports, psychiatrists can improve the complex neurodevelopmental issues in these individuals.

Medications may have positive or negative outcomes as patients with FASD are more sensitive to the CNS effects of medications.

i.   For example, selective serotonin reuptake inhibitors (SSRI's) such as fluoxetine, paroxetine, or citalopram, used not infrequently in Autism, may be more likely to precipitate agitation, activation, or suicidality in these brain- damaged adolescents due to augmentation of a pre-existing, organically-driven impulsivity.

At the same time, given that individuals with FASD may have deficiencies and/or differences in neurotransmitter systems such as serotonin and dopamine, low doses of sertraline and fluoxetine have proven anecdotally beneficial for some patients

ii.   Adolescents and young adults with ARND and co-occurring seizure disorders have a prenatally kindled organic brain dysfunction as a result of alcohol-induced damage to the corpus callosum, cerebellum or hippocampus. There is anecdotal clinical evidence that antiepileptics (i.e., carbamazepine, valproic acid, lamotrigine, neurontin) can be effective in preventing this kindling effect. The prenatal effects of alcohol can also result in a change in the balance of the developing neurotransmitters. Animal research has shown that prenatal alcohol can induce decrease in inhibitory neurotransmitter GABA in the hippocampus, and this neurochemical imbalance can underpin development of seizures (Hannigan et al 1996, Riley et al 2006). The effects of antiepileptics should be weighed carefully since some medications for seizures may also increase anxiety, affective/mood liability, and reduce learning and cognition.

4.4.5. The future for medication use in FASD including those with common presentations of ADHD, mood disorders and/or autism

i.   Obviously multicenter, randomized controlled clinical trials (ideally international) are needed in this vulnerable and clinically complex population. (Turk 2009)

ii.   There is a need for scientific testing and evaluation of new clinical instruments which combine cognitive, language, and behavioral response as the 'gold standard' for assessing medication efficacy and safety in patients with FASD. Currently there are no validated clinical instruments to evaluate the developmental, cognitive, language and behavioral response of a patient with FAS or ARND to psychotropic medication. There is a non-specific neuropsychiatric rating scale, but most drug rating scales (with the exception of those used in Alzheimer's disorder) evaluate clinical symptoms related to psychiatric disorder (i.e., Connor's Questionnaire, Beck Depression Inventory, Hamilton Rating Scale, CBCL).

iii.   It is long recognized that the use of multiple psychotropic medications is a risk for toxicity and acute confusional state, even in absence of underlying neurocognitive problems. The mechanism of multidrug interaction leading to toxicity relates to individual drugs competing for absorption through the liver cytochrome P450 2D6 enzyme system. In turn, certain medication blood levels increase (i.e., paroxetine is well known to increase blood levels of other psychotropic medications). In a recent lecture at the First European Conference on FASD in Rolduc, Holland (Nov 3rd to 5th 2010), Ken Warren, Acting Director of NIAAA, mentioned concern about medication interactions, but no data was given or studies forthcoming.

5. Discussion

This chapter has attempted to highlight the overlapping clinic al presentations of patients with FASD, whether dysmorphic FAS or non –dysmorphic ARND. Autism and Aspergers Disorder probably rank next to ADHD as the commonest clinical phenotype of FASD.

The lack of DSM or ICD Axis I codes for these individuals means that treating psychiatrists do not usually identify either disorder (dysmorphic or nondysmorphic conditions related to prenatal alcohol exposure as aetiological factors to be considered in diagnosis. The organic brain hypothesis will then inform management at many levels.

Nevertheless, the arrival of DSM V will hopefully herald new diagnostic categories which will capture more correctly some of these patients with FASD who show what are deemed ';autistic' features. Two proposed diagnostic categories, Social Communication Disorder and Alcohol Related Neurobiological Disorder are in serious consideration. It is hoped that Alcohol Related Neurodevelopmental Disorder (ARND), already well recognized, will replace the new category it more correctly captures the essence of the developmental psychiatric disorder (DSM 5 Symposium 2012).

Currently the generic "treatment as usual" prevents individuals with FASD from receiving appropriate multisystem and multimodal services, and further results in predictably poor outcomes for affected individuals and ultimately costly consequences for communities.

Brain imaging such as MRI, fMRI or SPECT scans studies may begin to map more specific areas of brain dysfunction related to prenatal alcohol exposure and psychiatric clinical presentation (Riley, et al 2005, Kodituwakku et al 2011, Coles et al 2011). Historically our scientific knowledge of damaged or diseased brain structure associated with infections such as syphilis, AIDS or lesions associated with cerebrovascular accidents has informed our diagnostic accuracy and informed treatment progress. Therefore it is not unrealistic to expect that correlations between the structural and functional deficits in individuals exposed at certain points during pregnancy could dramatically improve our understanding of brain function.

Finally, the ability to distinguish FASD with an autistic clinical presentation from a genetically-acquired or non-organic cause of this neurodevelopmental condition. This aetiological knowledge ultimately better describes the pathophysiology and neuropsychiatric phenomenology of the patient's clinical diagnosis. The neurodevelopmental clinical frame expands the clinician's understanding that the autistic presentation is actually a phenotype form of this specific acquired brain injury, The prenatal alcohol exposure creates a chemical, structural, and even electrical CNS environment that is "hard wired" very different from the other aetiological pathways for autism. The child or adolescent psychiatrist (ideally trained in developmental psychiatry) has a long recognized central role as the "case supervisor" for patients with patients with FASD, and is in the better position to manage the unfolding and clarification of the neurodevelopmental formulation, differential diagnosis, psychiatric co-morbidities, and psychopharmacology. Increased understanding of these complex patients through a neurodevelopment formulation, unraveling such issues as the hidden aetiology to the autism presentation will improve holistic clinical outcomes including the appropriate, targeted use of medication by the treating child/adolescent psychiatrists.

Author details

Kieran D. O'Malley
Charlemont Clinic/ Our Lady's Children's Hospital Crumlin, Dublin, Ireland

References

[1] Baren Cohen S, Ring, HA, Ballimore ET, Wheelwright, S,Ashwin C, Williams SCR (2000). The amygydala theory of autism. Neuroscience and Biobehavioural Reviews. , 24, 3355-3344.

[2] Blumstein, A, Farrington, D. O, & Mortea, S. D. (1985). Delinquent Careers: Innocence, Desistance and Persistence in an Annual Review of Research, , 6

[3] Bonthius, D, Woodhopuse, J, Bonthius, N. E, Taggrad, D. A, & Lothman, E. W. (2001). Reduced seizure control and hippocampal cell loss in rats exposed to alcohol during brain growth spurt. Alcohol Exp Clin Res., 25, (1) 70-82

[4] Bookstein, F. L, Sampson, P. D, Streissguth, A. P, & Connor, P. L. (2001). Geometric morphometrics of corpus callosum and subcortical structures in fetal alcohol effected brain. Teratology: , 4, 4-32.

[5] British Medical Association Board of Science (2007). Fetal Alcohol Spectrum Disorders: A Guide for Professionals. Publisher: BMA, London.

[6] Byrne, C. (2008). April). Psychopharmacology Basics for FASD. Workshop Presentation, 3rd Biennial Conference Adolescents and Adults with FASD. Vancouver, Canada.

[7] Carpenter, B. (2012). st Intercountry Adoption Conference, Plenary Talk, Education Issues in FASD, Cork, Jan 21st

[8] CDCFAS: Guidelines for Referral and Diagnosis (CDC, HHS, NOFAS, (2005). th Printing. National Center Birth Defects and Developmental Disabilities, Centers for Disease Control and Prevention, Department of Health Human Services, and NOFAS, USA.

[9] Chess, S. (1971). Autism in children with congenital Rubella. Journal of Autism and Developmental Disorders. 1(1), 33-47

[10] Clarren, S. K, & Smith, D. W. (1978). The Fetal Alcohol Syndrome: A review of the world literature. New England Journal of Medicine. , 298, 1063-1067.

[11] Clarren, S. K, Astley, S. J, & Bowden, D. M. (1988). Physical Anomalies and Developmental Delays in Nonhuman Primate Infants Exposed to Weekly Doses of Ethanol During Gestation. Teratology , 37, 561-569.

[12] Chudley, A. E, Conry, J, Cook, J. L, Loock, C, & Rosales, T. le Blanc N ((2005). March 1) Fetal Alcohol Spectrum Disorder: Canadian Guideline for Diagnosis. Can. Med. Assoc. Journal, 172 (5 supplement).

[13] Coles, C. (2009). IHE Consensus Developmental Conference. FASD: Across the Lifespan. Management Strategies. Westin Hotel, Edmonton, Alberta, Canada.

[14] Coles CD & Zhihao L ((2011). Functional neuroimaging in the examination of effects of prenatal alcohol exposureNeuropsychology Review, in press.

[15] Cummings, E. M, Davies, P. T, & Campbell, S. B. (2000). developmental psychopathology and Family Process. Theory,Research and Clinical Implications. The Guilford Press, London, New York.

[16] DSM 5 Symposium ((2012). The making of DSM S. Part 1. AACAP, 59th annual meeting Oct 25th, San Francisco..

[17] Elias, S. E, Coughlan, B. J, & O'Malley, KD. (2012). Fetal alcohol spectrum disorders: children, parents and carers of living with the disorder: a mixed methods approach, Poster Presentation SSBP International Conference, Leuven Belgium, Oct 10th to 12th

[18] Fitzgerald, M. (2010). Violent and Dangerous to Know. Nova Science Publishers, New York. Available at www.amazon.com.

[19] Gardner H Spiegelman DBaka S ((2011). Perinatal and neonatal risk factors for autism: A comprehensive meta analysis. Pediatrics, , 128(2)

[20] Gilberg, C, & Gilberg, C. I. (1983). Infantile autism. A total population study of reduced optimality in the pre, peri and neonatal period. Journal of Autism and Developmental Disorders, t, 32(4), 153-166.

[21] Glancy, G. D, & Knott, T. F. Part I: the Psychopharmacology of Long-Term Aggression-Toward an Evidence-Based Algorithm. Canadian Psychiatric Association Bulletin, Psychiatry and the Law.

[22] Glancy, G. D, & Knott, T. F. Part II: The Psychopharmacology of Long-Term Aggression-Toward an Evidence-Based Algorithm, Canadian Psychiatric Association Bulletin. Psychiatry and the Law.

[23] Greene, T, Ernhardt, C. B, Ager, J, Sokol, R, Martier, S, & Boyd, T. (1991). Prenatal Alcohol Exposure and Cognitive Development in the Preschool Years. Neurotoxicology and Teratology, , 13, 57-68.

[24] Hagerman, R. J. (1999). Neurodevelopmental Disorders. Diagnosis and Treatment. Oxford University Press, New York, Oxford., 3-47.

[25] Hannigan, J, & Randall, S. (1996). Behavioural pharmacology in animals exposed prenatally to alcohol. In Abel, EL, editor, Fetal alcohol syndrome. From mechanism to prevention. CRC Press, New York,, 191-213.

[26] Hobson, R. P. (1989). Beyond Cognition. A theory of autism. In Dawson G, ed,.Autism, nature, diagnosis and treatment. Guilford Press, New York,, 222-448.

[27] Hosenbocus, S, & Chahal, R. (2012). a review of executive function deficits and paharmacological management in children and adolescents. J can acad. Child adolesc. Psychaitry, 21, (3)

[28] National Institute on Alcohol Abuse and Alcoholism (NIAAA (2000). June). Highlights from Current Research: 10th Special Report to the U.S. Congress on Alcohol and Health from the Secretary of Health and Human Services. US Department of Health and Human Services, Public Health Service, National Institutes of Health.

[29] Jones, K. L, & Smith, D. W. (1973). Recognition of the Fetal Alcohol Syndrome in early infancy, Lancet, , 2, 999-1001.

[30] Jones, K. L, & Smith, D. W. (1975). The Fetal Alcohol Syndrome, Teratology, 1975,12: 1-10.

[31] Kodituwaddu FW & Koditowakku EL ((2011). From research to practiceAn integrative framework for the development of interventions in children with featl alcohol spectrum disorders. Neuropsychology Review, , 21, 204-223.

[32] Lee, R, & Coccaro, E. (2001). Feb) The Neuropsychopharmacology of Criminality and Aggression. Canadian Journal of Psychiatry, , 46

[33] LemoineP Harousseau H, Borteyru JP ((1968). Les infants de parents alcoholi-ques.Anomalies observes a propos de 127 cas. Quest Med. , 21, 476-482.

[34] Lord, C. Mulloy, C Wendelboe M., Schopler E((1991). Pre and perinatal factors in high functioning females and males with autism. J autism Dev Disorder, , 21(2), 197-209.

[35] Lord C Kim SHDimartino A ((2011). Autism Spectrum Disorders. General Overview. Chapter 14, Editors Howlin P, Charman T, Ghaziuddin M, The Sage Handbook of Developmental Disorders, Published London, California, New Delhi, Singapore

[36] Mukarjee, R, Hollins, S, & Turk, J. (2006). Psychiatric comorbidity in fetal alcohol syndrome. Psychiatric Bulletin. , 30, 194-195.

[37] Mukarjee, R, Hollins, S, & Curfs, L. (2012). Fetal Alcohol Spectrum Disorders. Is it something we should be more aware of? J R Coll.Physicians, Edin. 21, 2, 42, 143-150

[38] Nanson, J. (1991). Autism in Fetal Alcohol Syndrome. A report of 6 cases. Alcoholism. Clinical and Experimental Research

[39] Novick BrownN, O'Malley, KD, Streissguth, AP ((2010). FASD: Diagnostic Dilemmas and Challenges for a Modern Transgenerational Management Approach. In Editors, Abubado, S, Cohen D, Prenatal Alcohol Use and Fetal Alcohol Spectrum Disorders: A Model Standard of Diagnosis, Assessment and Multimodal Treatment, Bentham Online Publishing, USA.

[40] O'Malley, K. D, & Barr, HM. (1998). Fetal Alcohol Syndrome and Seizure Disorder. Letter to editor, Can J Psychiatry.

[41] O'Malley, K. D, & Storoz, L. (2003). Fetal Alcohol Spectrum Disorder and ADHD. Diagnostic implications and therapeutic consequences. Expert Review of Neurotherapeutics. , 3(4)

[42] O'Malley, K. D. (2008). (Ed.) ADHD and Fetal Alcohol Spectrum Disorders. 2nd Printing, Nova Science Publishers, New York., CHAPTERS 1, 4, 6, 11

[43] O'Malley, K. D. (2010). Fetal Alcohol Spectrum Disorders. in Enyclopedia of Psychopharmacolgy, Springer-Verlag, Berlin, Heidelberg.

[44] O'Malley, K. D, & Mukarjee, R. (2010). Fetal Alcohol Stndrome, Alcohol Related Neurodevelopmental Disorder, Syndrome Phenotypes, Society Study of Behavioural Phenotypes, UK,www.ssbp.co.uk

[45] O'Malley, K. D. (2011a). ADHD and FASD. From animal research to clinical experience. Invited talk, International CADDRA meeting Toronto, October 16th

[46] O'Malley, K. D. (2011b). Fetal Alcohol Spectrum Disorders. Chapter The Sage Handbook of Devevelopmental Disorders. Howlin P, Charman T, Ghazziuddin M, Editors. Published, London, California, New Delhi, Singapore, 24, 479-496.

[47] Orphan Drug ActUS Congress; Designation of Drugs for Rare Diseases or Conditions; SEC. 526 [360bb]. (a)(1)

[48] Pennington, B. F. (2009). Diagnosing Learning Disorders. A Neuropsychological Framework. 2nd Edition, The Guilford Press, London, New York

[49] Rich, S. D. (2005). Fetal Alcohol Syndrome: Preventable Tragedy. Psychiatric News, Residents' Forum. Page 12., 40(9)

[50] Rich, S. D, Sulik, K. K, Jones, K. L, Riley, E. P, & Chambers, C. (2009). Nov). Fetal Alcohol Spectrum Disorder: A Paradigm for Neurodevelopmental Formulation and Multidisciplinary Treatment. Presented at the American Academy of Child and Adolescent Psychiatry Annual Conference, Honolulu, Hawaii.

[51] Rich SD & O'Malley KD (2012). A neurodevelopmental formulation for the psychiatric care of Fetal Alcohol Spectrum Disorders. Journal of psychiatry and the Law, Accepted.

[52] Riley, E. P, & Mcgee, C. L. (2005). Fetal Alcohol Spectrum Disorders: an overview with emphasis on changes in brain and behavior. Experimental Biology and Medicine, , 230, 357-365.

[53] Russell, J. (1997). Autism is an executive disorder. Oxford University Press, New York

[54] Sokol, R. J, Delaney-black, V, & Nordstrom, B. (2003). Dec 10). Fetal Alcohol Spectrum Disorder JAMA, , 290(22)

[55] Solomon, M, Hessl, D, Chiu, S, Olsen, E, & Hendren, R. (2009). March 1). Towards a Neurodevelopmental Model of Clinical Case Formulation., Psychiatric Clinics of North America. , 32(1), 199-211.

[56] Stratton, K, Howe, C, & Battaglia, F. (1996). Fetal Alcohol Syndrome. Diagnosis, Epidemiology, Prevention, and Treatment, Institute of Medicine, National Academy Press, Washington DC, USA.

[57] Steinhausen, H-C, Willms, J, & Spohr, H-L. (1993). Sept). Long-Term Psychophathological and Cognitive Outcome of Children with Fetal Alcohol Syndrome. Journal of the American Academy of Child and Adolescent Psychiatry, 32:5, , 990-994.

[58] Streissguth, A. P, Aase, J. M, Clarren, S. K, & Randels, S. P. LaDue RA, Smith DF ((1991). April 17). Fetal Alcohol Syndrome in Adolescents and Adults, Journal of the American Medical Association, , 265(15), 1966.

[59] Streissguth, A. P. and LaDue RA ((1987). Fetal Alcohol Teratogenic Causes of Developmental Disabilities. In S. Schroeder (Ed.), Toxic Substances and Mental Retardation, Washington, DC: American Association on Mental Deficiency, , 1-32.

[60] Streissguth, A. P, Barr, H. M, Kogan, J, & Bookstein, F. L. (1996). Understanding the occurrence of secondary disabilities in clients with fetal alcohol syndrome (FAS) and fetal alcohol effects(FAE) Final Report CDC Grant R04, USA

[61] Streissguth AP & O'Malley KD ((2000). Neuropsychiatric Implications and Long Term Psychiatric Consequences of Fetal Alcohol Spectrum DisordersSeminars in Clinical Neuropsychiatry, , 5(3)

[62] Sulik, K. K, Johnston, M. C, & Webb, M. A. (1983). Fetal Alcohol Syndrome: Embryogenesis in a Mouse Model. Science, , 214, 936-38.

[63] Turk, J. (2009). Behavioural Phenotypes in Relation to ADHD. ADHD in Practice. UK., 1(3)

[64] Turk, J. (2012). Behavioural Phenotypes. Royal College of Learning Disability Psychiatrists residential meeting, Manchester, Sepember 27th

[65] Vocci, F. J, Acri, J, & Elksahef, A. (2005). Medication Development for Addictive Disorders: The State of The Science. Am J. Psychiatry, , 162(8), 1432-1440.

[66] US Surgeon General (2005, Feb 21). U.S. Surgeon General Releases Advisory on Alcohol Use in Pregnancy: Urges women who are pregnant or who may become pregnant to abstain from alcohol. http://www.surgeongeneral.gov/pressreleases/sg02222005.html. US Department of Health and Human Services, Office of the Surgeon General.

[67] Bonnin A ,Goedein N ,Chen K, Wilson ML, King J, Shih JC, Blakely RD, Deneris ES, Levitt P (2011) A transient placental source of serotonin for fetal forebrain. Nature, April

Aetiological Factors - Parents and Families

Chapter 6

Empowering Families in the Treatment of Autism

Jennifer Elder

Additional information is available at the end of the chapter

1. Introduction

It is well known that autism is a complex, currently incurable disorder with an unclear etiology, and that individuals with autism typically have normal life expectancies which require parents, and later siblings, to provide varying levels of lifelong care. Because of the complexity of the disease, it is critically important to help families understand the disorder, manage stress, and sift through information that frequently includes erroneous media views and unsubstantiated claims of treatment efficacy. This chapter will help families and advising professionals by providing them with an overview of several topics: first, the common reactions and beliefs about autism and individuals with autism that are held by family members; second, the family-centered as well as complementary and alternative treatment approaches that are currently available; and finally, the best recommendations for helping families adapt to an autism diagnosis and maintain healthy functioning as caregivers—all while planning for, and addressing the lifelong needs of, individuals with autism.

2. Common reactions and beliefs held by family members

Families are faced with enormous challenges in caring for children with autism over a lifetime. The first challenge is obtaining the initial diagnosis, which can be difficult despite the fact that autism is better understood today than it was in the past. Indeed, it is common for families to consult a variety of professionals such as pediatricians and primary health care providers before receiving a conclusive diagnosis. Once the diagnosis is made, however, parents face a second, far greater challenge: mourning the loss of their "perfect child"—which can be a long and arduous process that involves coming to terms with the fact that their child, whose physical appearance is normal or even unusually attractive, has a complex, incurable, and frequently debilitating condition. After the family advances through stages of grieving that can be characterized using Elizabeth Kübler-Ross's five stages of grief—Denial, Anger, Bargaining, Depression, and Acceptance (DABDA)—they eventually arrive at a "new normal" with family harmony reestablished [1].

The first stage of grieving, denial, is common in parents of children with autism, and can persist even after a child receives a diagnosis. Because fathers are typically less involved in day-to-day care than mothers, they may experience denial more intensely due to fewer opportunities to observe the symptoms. For example, a father may be more likely to say, "he doesn't have autism; he's just quiet," which is supported by stories of other family members who were also "late to develop" yet still "turned out fine". However, as the symptoms of autism become more conspicuous, caregivers notice differences between their child and other, typically developing children whom they encounter in playgrounds, preschools, and family gatherings. Frequently, it is extended family members who identify the autistic symptoms, share their concerns with the primary caregivers and try to convince the caretakers to seek further assessment and follow up as needed. This action is critical to accurate and timely diagnosis, early intervention (< age 3), and improved prognosis for overall quality of life.

The next stage, "anger", may result in family members asking "Why us?" or "Why did this have to happen to him?" During this time, family tension is high and anger may also be expressed toward intervening professionals, especially if there has been a prior lack of, or slow responsiveness to, parental concerns. For example, one parent stated, "That pediatrician should have listened to me when I expressed concern about David not speaking at four years old; instead, he told me not to worry about it." This failure to identify the signs sooner can lead to destructive self-blame, resulting in self-talk such as, "If only I had recognized the signs sooner" or "I knew we should have sought other opinions"—comments that may be responded to with active listening (e.g. "You sound as though you are experiencing a lot of regret") and nonjudgmental advice (e.g. "Many parents struggle at this time. What is important is that you are seeking the necessary assistance now.") In addition to self-blame related to behavior, it is also common in this stage for parents to evaluate their genealogy to determine who was genetically responsible for the disorder. Unfortunately, there is no conclusive genetic test for autism and while genetics likely plays a role, environmental factors may also contribute to its development.

The third stage, "bargaining", can place families at great risk because it involves frantically seeking ways to reverse the diagnosis even if those ways are implausible. For example, it is common for parents to directly bargain with a higher power (e.g. "If you cure my child, I will be a better parent") or indirectly, with a lesser power such as the health care profession (e.g. If I find the "right" doctor or medication, my child will be cured). As they desperately seek a "magic bullet", parents may interrogate health care providers about the most useful medications despite the fact that no single medication is effective for all symptoms. In addition, parents may surf the Internet and read testimonials regarding treatments that are not empirically sound; consequently, well-informed professionals need to advise families against these treatments as some are risky and can lead to financial burden. (The most common treatment approaches will be described later in this chapter.)

The fourth stage, "depression", can take many forms. Parents may at times feel over-whelmed and powerless in their ability to facilitate their child's development or ameliorate difficult, disruptive behaviors such as severe tantrums or self-abuse. Indeed, negative be-haviors may intensify to such a degree that families curtail their usual plans or avoid a de-sired activity all together, leading to feelings of hopelessness that is expressed in statements such as, "I can't do anything right" or "why bother". In addition, because many children with autism have sleep disturbances (e.g., difficulty falling asleep; waking up and becoming active in the middle of the night), parents must be vigilant at night, causing exhaustion and sometimes even deeper depression. At this point, it is important for caregivers to recognize that they may need professional help such as counseling or prescribed medications in order to optimally provide for their child and family.

Many families who advance to acceptance, the final stage, describe having gained spiritual strength, which helped them maintain "hope"—an essential ingredient to successful griev-ing. In this stage, families recognize that there is no instant cure for their child's autism, but there are credible interventions that can help. Ultimately, families discover that they can be powerful advocates for their children, and after receiving proper education, can implement home interventions that positively affect the family unit and even improve their child's con-dition. Once they gain confidence in these new approaches, they can serve other families struggling through the grieving process by contributing empathy and wisdom to local fami-ly support group meetings. Because grieving is rarely a linear process, these meetings can also help families as they revisit earlier stages by limiting the time they spend in previous ones, thus facilitating a more permanent acceptance.

3. Families as primary interveners

3.1. Parent training

Historically, development of more family-focused interventions has resulted in a shift from didactic teaching and family therapy models to interactive approaches, in which parents are active participants in all levels of the training process [2, 3]. Although parents were once viewed as the cause of their child's problems [4-6], they are now recognized for the key roles they can play in ongoing child training and skill generalization [7-9], which has led to better child prognosis and long-term quality of life.

Because there are now clearer linkages between core constructs such as *social reciprocity* (e.g. social turn-taking), *joint attention* (e.g. sharing interest in, and mutually commenting on, an object), and language acquisition, developing these skills can improve a child's communica-tive capacity. In fact, researchers stress that teaching parents to target pivotal skills such as joint attention may produce positive, sustained effects on social and language development [10]. Similarly, evidence suggests that interventions that require parents to synchronize with the child's attentional focus (i.e. become interested in what the child is interested in) may be more effective than parent-directed approaches (e.g., instructing the child to play with a toy in a certain way) for children who have difficulty responding to, or initiating, joint attention

[11]. However, there is a need to closely examine the individual parent-training intervention components thought to be linked with these core constructs to determine which components are most effective for a particular child. This would allow researchers to better identify the most convenient and efficient means of teaching these constructs and related intervention components.

3.2. Research development in parent training

The author and co-investigators have been following a systematic sequence of research that began in the early 1980's with the development of a play-based, in-home intervention that was initially tested in-depth, over 8-12 weeks, with four mother-child dyads using intrasubject (single subject experimental) methodology [12]. In this initial study, Elder found that mothers figure prominently as recipients of training and other interventions and that even when the focus was on the dyad, mothers "took over" and fathers stayed in the "background," with inadequate diffusion of new learning through the mothers. This lack of father involvement piqued the interest of Elder's research team, who collaborated on new studies directed at fathers. Although a systematic review of the literature revealed only three intervention studies that included fathers, evidence indicated that fathers' interaction styles differed from mothers, possibly resulting in unique contributions to their child's social and language development [13].

Building on Lamb's (1987) seminal work related to fathers and their influence on child development, Elder et al. developed and tested a Father Directed In-Home Training (FDIT) intervention with a total of 36 father-child and mother-child dyads under controlled conditions in two NIH/NINR-funded studies [7, 8]. The study was designed so that data from individual training components could be analyzed rather than an entire intervention package. These training components were based on the theoretical constructs in social interaction theory and characterized by the broad concept of social "turn-taking". Because the team had previously observed many fathers sitting passively or aggressively directing interactions and not allowing their child time to respond, the research team created four intervention components: (a) following the child's lead (FCL), which involved allowing the child with autism to direct play, (b) imitating/animating (I/A), which entailed attending to and imitating the ADS child's sounds and/or actions in an animated manner, (c) expectant waiting (E/W), which required signaling the child and waiting for a response, and (d) commenting on the child (CC), which emphasized remarking on the child's actions at appropriate times during play [12]. Fathers were instructed to watch videotaped examples and read written directions about integrating these components into play sessions. After mastering the skills, fathers taught mothers the same techniques using the research team's educational approach, resulting in both parents reporting that training had helped them relax during the in-home play sessions.

After the intervention, fathers significantly increased their use of the skills taught and children with autism responded with greatly increased initiating rates as well as frequencies of child non-speech vocalizations. In follow-up interviews, fathers revealed that the training had enhanced their paternal role and the quality of overall family functioning [14]. (Details of these studies can be found in published articles [7, 8]).

3.3. Including siblings

Most children with autism have difficulty with inconsistency as evidenced by their strong adherence to routines and rituals. Therefore, it may be difficult, perhaps even impossible, for these children to effectively modify their interactions if family members are not consistent in their approach. Furthermore, incongruence within the family can distress children with autism, who may express their feelings by engaging in a variety of aberrant behaviors such as tantrums, aggression, and other behavioral expressions of frustration. Present research indicates that training non-affected, typically developing siblings, or other individuals who have ongoing contact with the child with autism, could be beneficial. However, little is known about the effects of training siblings to use theoretically-derived strategies such as those Elder and others have implemented with parents. Also unknown is the effect that training typically developing siblings might have on their own behavior, anxiety, and overall quality of life. Although it seems likely that training would positively affect them, training effects on siblings should be addressed in clinical trials.

In a search of the literature related to non-affected, typically developing (TD) siblings of children with autism, few studies are found describing these children, their relationship with their sibling with autism, or what effect having a sibling with autism has on them [15]. Of the extant reports, the findings are inconsistent, making it difficult to characterize the siblings, identify those who are vulnerable to poor adjustment outcomes, or develop interventions that benefit both the sibling and the entire family [15]. It is clear, however, from both the literature and clinical experience, that TD siblings are often faced with unique challenges related to their affected sibling's autism. Also, because children with ADS rarely have physical disfigurement, it is often difficult for those who are not familiar with autism to understand why these children act the way they do; this, in turn, adds to the stress that TD siblings and the family experience [16-18]. Initial findings are promising because they show that when TD siblings care for their ADS siblings early in life, this can positively affect not only the child with autism but also the intervening sibling [19-22]. This clearly indicates that training and evaluating siblings is an area of research with enormous potential and clinical relevance.

Another important consideration that lends support for training siblings is evidence that children with autism learn best in naturalistic environments such as their homes. In a classic work, Baer, Wolf, and Risley (1968) state that skills taught to children in one setting cannot be expected to generalize to other settings without planned, systematic implementation. In fact, these researchers assert that no deliberate behavior changes, particularly related to language acquisition and socialization, should be made that are not reinforced regularly in the child's primary environment; otherwise, trainers must continue to intervene to maintain the behavior change [23]. If one ascribes to this view, clinic-taught interventions cannot be expected to generalize well to home settings unless: (a) the trainer is always present (an impractical and costly idea), (b) family members are taught to assist with generalization, or (c) ideally, intervening family members and children with autism are trained in familiar home environments where naturally reinforcing (caregiving) activities are more likely to occur. Also, children with autism are more likely to exhibit abnormal language in unfamiliar settings than at home [11]. For these reasons, it is important that AD children acquire communication skills in naturalistic settings where they are most likely to encounter interactions and opportunities to utilize communication skills that are similar to the contexts of their daily routines [11].

4. Using new technologies to train families

The use of the Internet has grown substantially over the last few years, with an estimated 260 million people now online in North America [24]. In addition, between 2000 and 2010 the proportion of Internet users who are black or Latino has nearly doubled, causing the Internet population to closely resemble the racial composition of the nation as a whole. Health information is one of the most important subjects researched online, and this is reflected in the autism community, where many families are heavily dependent upon Internet services for education, updates on autism treatment, and peer support via parent chat rooms [15].

However, despite the great interest in using the Internet as a resource for learning about autism, online parent training interventions are rare. Recently, considerable evidence has become available demonstrating that web-based feedback systems may increasingly provide feasible and cost-effective patient education [25] because they are available 24 hours a day and can be used repeatedly to enhance learning. Further, with wide-spread internet technology, it may now be possible to provide much needed training to families living remotely and to those representing previously underserved minorities. Clearly, there is an urgent need for clinicians and researchers who have manualized training interventions to adapt them for online use and systematically evaluate their effectiveness through clinical trials.

5. Managing family stress

Until the 1980's, the diagnosis of autism was generally not well-known and most children diagnosed with autism were eventually institutionalized. Today, the majority of these children live with their families, who face enormous challenges in planning for and providing a lifetime of care. Families often experience significant financial burden [26], insecurity regarding long-term family planning, and stress related to the child's social impairments and adverse behaviors that often interfere with family functioning [27, 28]. Because additional care giving has been shown to predict parental distress [29] and parents of children with autism may experience greater stress than parents of children with other disabilities, interventions and techniques that can reduce stress are needed [30-34].

Although caring for a child with ASD can adversely affect quality of life for both parents [35], most research related to parental stress has focused on mothers [36] who have reported higher stress levels than fathers [31, 37-40]. However, in two other studies comparing mothers' and fathers' stress levels, no differences were found [32, 41]. The author and team also found that both mothers and fathers scored very high, over the 90th percentile on the Parenting Stress Index pre-intervention with no statistical significance between the mothers' and fathers' scores [14].

In 2008, Davis and Carter provided more insight regarding how mothers and fathers may react to their child's autism. They noted that although mothers had a higher rate of stress and depression, fathers reported more difficulty interacting with the children. In addition, mothers were more involved with everyday activities and thus, more often affected by their child's inability to perform activities of daily living and self-regulate emotions. In contrast, fathers reacted more to overt behaviors such as tantrums, aggression, and/or loud/peculiar vocalizations, which are particularly difficult to manage and can be embarrassing in public settings. Because the core disability associated with autism is social, it can be stressful for parents to deal with a child who may not like to be held, will not respond to their affection, or even make eye contact.

Although only a few studies have explored effects of child intervention on changes in parental stress levels, [14, 28, 42, 43] results are promising. Parent involvement that results in improved child outcomes can empower parents and lower stress in both mothers and fathers. Also, it is important to consider that although fathers may not appear to be as overtly stressed as mothers, there is evidence that they also experience high levels of stress; therefore, interventions should include both mothers and fathers. Finally, although little is known about stress in siblings, it is likely that their stress is also high and that they could benefit from being included in an intervention.

6. Alternative and complementary therapies: Helping families

6.1. Select credible treatment options

A report from the American Academy of Pediatrics' Council on Children with Disabilities states that treatment goals for children with autism are to: (a) maximize the child's ultimate functional independence and quality of life by minimizing the core features, (b) facilitate development and learning, (c) promote socialization, (d) reduce maladaptive behaviors, and (e) educate and support families [44]. While standard treatments meet these goals and thus, are generally accepted by the autism research community, the variety of novel approaches are less accepted due to their lack of empirical support. As a result, families, who often become desperate to identify a ready cure for the disorder, must be equipped with the knowledge to avoid scams by fully evaluating the potential of new therapeutic approaches.

While it is not possible to cover the multitude of novel and complementary treatments for autism, the author will provide a critical review of some of the most popular strategies, ferreting out those that are empirically validated from those that are unsubstantiated. This section will include a discussion of findings from the author's previously published, randomized clinical trial that evaluated the effects of the popular Gluten-Free, Casein-Free diet on individuals with autism, and subsequently recommend directions for future research.

6.2. Dietary intervention and nutritional supplements in autism

Increasingly, parents are using alternative treatments, such as dietary interventions or supplements, which they learn about from internet sites or anecdotal reports from other parents. Perhaps the most well-known dietary intervention is the gluten-free casein-free (GFCF) diet that restricts consumption of wheat and dairy products, and which adherents claim can "cure" autism [45]. This diet is so popular that a person can simply type, "GFCF" and "autism" into Google's search engine, and hundreds of sites appear—from the "Gluten-Free Trading Co." to "GFCF Diet Success Stories" with endorsements such as the following: "Three weeks ago, I decided to give it [GFCF diet] a try. After three days without dairy, Wow! Suddenly we had an alert child! He was talking more, making sense of the world, and engaging with us! When I phased out wheat and gluten, he got even better. He is happier; his behavior is better; his muscle tone seems to be improving; his eye contact is great; he is speaking like a normal 4 year old!" [46] Although testimonies like these abound on the Internet, there is limited empirical data to support the claims, resulting in a lack of data that health care providers can use to effectively guide parents in making informed decisions.

This dietary intervention, which has clearly "raced ahead of science," poses health risks as well as financial and social drawbacks. While it is less costly than when it was originally introduced, the GFCF diet can still add financial strain to families and may even compromise nutritional health (e.g., insufficient calcium) in children with autism who already have restricted food repertoires. There are also social costs to the children, who cannot eat foods unless they are prepared at home, ruling out the possibility of eating cake, for example, at a birthday party. Similarly, families experience a social cost because they have to prepare dual meals plans that often consist of time-consuming recipes. Thus, unless families have additional financial or social assistance, the GFCF diet can represent a significant burden to a family already struggling with caring for a child with autism.

Despite the continuing popularity of this diet, only five controlled studies have been published since 1999. Three of these studies—Knivsberg [47], Whiteley [48], and Johnson[49]—were not double-blind. That is, parents not only knew when their children were receiving the GFCF diet but were also responsible for implementing it. Of these three single blind studies, Knivsberg [47] and Whiteley [48] reported positive findings but have been criticized for their reliance on reports from parents who were not blinded to the dietary intervention. However, it should be noted that Knivsberg [47] conducted a year-long study and some proponents of the GFCF diet suggest that the short duration of other clinical trials may have been responsible for the insignificant findings.

The other two studies were double blind randomized control trials. In the first study, Elder [50] partnered with researchers and staff at the University of Florida's (UF) General Clinical Research Center [now part of UF's Clinical Translational Science Institute Research (CTSI)] to conduct the first double-blind placebo controlled clinical trial of the GFCF diet that was published in *The Journal of Autism and Developmental Disorders* (2006). The researchers evaluated the effects of the GFCF diet on: (a) autistic symptoms as measured by the Childhood Autism Rating Scale (CARS), Ecological Communication Orientation Scale (ECOS), and behavioral frequencies of child social and language behaviors, and (b) urinary peptide levels of gluten and casein. After videotaping the participating 13 children, aged 2 to 16 years, during in-home play sessions for 15 minutes before the diet's introduction, at the end of the first 6-week period, and at the completion of the 12-week protocol, Elder [50] found that group analysis showed no significant differences in any of the outcomes measured or urinary peptide levels of gluten and casein. Even when they were told that the findings were insignificant, parents of nine children kept the children on the diet, indicating that a strong "parent placebo effect" may exist and be responsible for perpetuating the diet's popularity.

In the second study by Hyman [51], children were given the GFCF diet and provided with food challenges; that is, snacks that contained gluten or casein, and which were disguised so that the participants could not identify if the snacks were GFCF. As in the other clinical trials, these investigators used a variety of well-established outcome measures but like Elder [50], found no significant differences or empirical support for the diet. Despite the insignificant findings, the GFCF diet continues to be popular with parents, leading to the author's published recommendations about how to properly advise families regarding diet: first, parents may use the GFCF diet as long as the child does not have a severely restricted food repertoire that could lead to a nutritional deficiency; and second, the family has the social and financial resources to continue the diet [7].

Similar to dietary interventions, nutritional supplements are frequently used by parents to to treat their child's symptoms although there is little sound empirical evidence to support their efficacy in autism. Vitamins C, D, and the B vitamins are generally known to improve immunity, brain function, and overall nervous system activity [52-55]. As a result, they are often included in special autism supplements, which are specifically blended to treat autism-related symptoms. Other supplements that are frequently used include probiotics and digestive enzymes, which may help treat gastrointestinal problems such as acid reflux and constipation, and melatonin, a natural sleep aid that may help reduce nighttime sleep disturbances [56]. Finally, Omega-3 fatty acids, which have been shown to enhance neurological health in the general population, are currently being evaluated in several clinical trials for the treatment of autism [57]. Despite the lack of empirical support for these supplements, most are generally considered harmless if administered in age-appropriate doses.

6.3. Other approaches

Because of speculation that oxygen flow to the brain is reduced in children with autism, "hyperbaric treatments," in which individuals with autism are placed in a chamber and exposed to very high oxygen levels, have become popular. In 2009, the US ABC news network broadcast a story, "The Search for a Cure" describing preliminary results from a trial by Dr. Daniel A. Rossignol, himself a father of two children with autism. He and his colleagues evaluated hyperbaric treatment in 56 children with varying degrees of autism ranging in age from 2 to 7 years [58, 59]. Reports were positive, indicating that 30 percent of the children who received the treatment had greatly increased functioning, while only 8 percent in the control group did. In response to this study, Paul Ott, a M.D., autism expert, and author of *Autism's False Prophets* commented on the questionable efficacy of the treatment and emphasize its potential to financially drain families [60]. For example, a one-hour treatment can cost $100 to $900, and generally at least 40 are recommended. Despite his warning, however, the ABC report concluded on an approving note by stating, "While its positive effects remain unclear, hyperbaric chamber therapy does not present the dangers that other therapies do," thus encouraging parents to consider using an unproven and expensive treatment.

Although hyperbaric treatments are one of the latest alternative therapies to become popular in the autism community, parents have long used other unsubstantiated, pharmaceutical approaches. For example, antibiotics have often been prescribed for children with autism who have frequent respiratory or gastrointestinal infections; similarly, antifungal agents, such as nystatin and fluconazole, have been prescribed for children who suffer from an overgrowth of gastrointestinal yeast (e.g. Candida) [61]. In both situations, the medications are prescribed due to the erroneous belief that an infection or "imbalance" is the root cause of the disorder. Other speculative treatments include the intravenous administration of secretin, a gastrointestinal hormone, and immunoglobulin-G, an immune system antibody, which are popular because of a few, uncontrolled studies that demonstrated improvement [62]. Despite their questionable efficacy—several gold standard clinical trials have invalidated the use of secretin—alternative treatments are high in demand, generating countless articles on the Internet, and sparking heated discussion on autism message boards [63]. This prevailing popularity, which shows no sign of slowing in the future, is a testament to the struggle many parents experience in caring for a child with autism.

Another popular, yet more controversial treatment is chelation therapy, which removes mercury—an alleged contributor to autism—from the body. When using this therapy, parents typically have a medical doctor treat their child for lead poisoning or they may also buy unregulated chelation agents from Internet sites. Unlike hyperbaric treatment and other interventions that are intended to complement evidence-based treatments, advocates of chelation therapy espouse it as a cure. Yet, to date, there is no proven link between mercury exposure and autism [64]. Joecker, a researcher from the Mayo Clinic warns that not only is chelation therapy's efficacy unproven, but also that it can be associated with serious side effects, including potentially deadly liver and kidney damage and as a result should be assiduously avoided [65].

7. Interventions with empirical validation

After the preceding discussion of popular yet largely unproven interventions, the author would be remiss not to provide at least a brief overview of interventions that are empirically sound. Because autism presentations can vary greatly among individuals, each intervention should be customized to meet the needs of the individual child, and be accompanied with the early speech/language and occupational therapy that are typically indicated.

In addition to the special education and pharmacological interventions that may be necessary, traditional treatment approaches include providing a child with speech, behavioral, occupational, and physical therapy as indicated in some cases. Although public schools in the United States are required by law to provide such services, the frequency, type, and quality of these services vary considerably. Consequently, parents need to actively participate in meetings where Individualized Educational Plans (IEP), or the equivalent, are developed to specifically address a child's behavioral or learning needs. Furthermore, parents should maintain close contact with educational personnel to help evaluate their children's progress and determine the future direction of treatment.

If the future direction includes medications, parents must carefully analyze the costs and benefits by questioning their health care provider regarding possible improvements and side effects. Although medications do not cure autism, sometimes they can alleviate behavioral symptoms that distress the child and interfere with therapeutic efforts such as intensive education and socialization [66-68]. These behavioral symptoms include hyperactivity, self-injury, aggression, compulsions (repetitive behaviors), mood lability, anxiety, and sleep disturbances [69].

In addition to medication, parents may consider using a behavioral intervention, which researchers have refined over time and developed into a highly successful treatment approach. In particular, two comprehensive behavioral early interventions—Lovaas' Model based on Applied Behavior Analysis (ABA) and the Early Start Denver Model—have been shown to be helpful in improving symptoms related to autism [70, 71]. Mounting evidence also supports the use of other commonly used therapies such as Floortime, Pivotal Response Therapy and Verbal Behavior Therapy [72-74]. For up-to-date information regarding behavioral interventions, visit the website for Autism Speaks, an internationally recognized organization within the autism community, at http://www.autismspeaks.org/what-autism/treatment. By visiting this site, parents will learn about the many valid treatments available that are safe, effective, and capable of producing a better quality of life for children with autism and their families.

8. Relationship of family training intervention research to NIH's priorities and NIMH's sponsored work-group recommendations

Finding ways to improve quality of life for ADS children and their families is one of the top priorities of NIH and congressionally mandated research as noted in the Combating Autism Act of 2006 [75, 76]. A report from a NIMH-supported work group of well-known autism authorities addresses what has traditionally been problematic in the field of autism [77]; namely, that fragmented and isolated individual study approaches have not been effective in systematically advancing the most effective behavioral interventions [78]. In response, Smith et al. proposed a developmental process for designing and conducting studies on psychosocial interventions in autism, which provides a way to systematically validate and disseminate interventions; the process includes the following steps: (a) conduct initial efficacy studies that may utilize intrasubject methodology to provide in-depth information about individual responses over time, (b) manualize the intervention and pilot-test it with larger numbers of participants, (c) conduct clinical trials to test the efficacy under controlled conditions, and (d) conduct effectiveness studies to evaluate outcomes in community settings.

The author and team have been following a developmental sequence that is consistent with that of the NIMH work group and especially part of the final step—evaluating outcomes in community settings. Delivering the training to all family members including siblings, and providing training interventions using state of the art internet technology would greatly expand our ability to deliver comprehensive family-centered training in the community, and produce significant gains that would improve the quality of life for individuals with autism and their families.

Author details

Jennifer Elder

Address all correspondence to: elderjh@ufl.edu

University of Florida College of Nursing, Gainesville, Florida, USA

References

[1] Ross EK-R, Kessler D. Finding the meaning of grief through the five stages of loss. New York: Scribner; 2007 2007. 256 p.

[2] Gross D, Fogg L, Tucker S. The efficacy of parent training for promoting positive parent-toddler relationships. Research in Nursing and Health. 1995;18(6):486-99.

[3] Webster-Stratton C, Herbert M. What really happens in parent-training? Behavior Modification. 1993;17:407-56.

[4] Bettelheim B. Feral Children and Autistic Children. american Journal of Sociology. 1959;64(5):455-7.

[5] Eisenberg L. THE FATHERS OF AUTISTIC CHILDREN*. American Journal of Orthopsychiatry. 1957;27(4):715-24.

[6] Kanner L. Autistic disturbances of affective contact. Nervous Child. 1943;2:217-50.

[7] Elder J, Donaldson S, Kairella J, Valcante G, Bendixen R, Ferdig RE, et al. In-home training for fathers of children with autism: A follow up study and evaluation of four individual training components. Journal of Child and Family Studies. 2010;20(3): 263-71.

[8] Elder J, Valcante G, Yarandi H, White D, Elder TH. Evaluating in-home training for fathers of children with autism using single-subject experiementation and group analysis methods. Nursing Research. 2005;54(1):22-32.

[9] Rogers SJ. Evidence-based interventions for language development in young children with autism. Social & communication development in autism spectrum disorders. T. S. Charman, W. ed. New York: Guildford Press; 2006. p. 143-79.

[10] Mundy P, Sigman M, Kasari C. A longitudinal study of joint attention and language development in autistic children. Journal of Autism and Developmental Disorders. 1990;20(1):115-28.

[11] Wetherby AM. Understanding and measuring social communication in children with autism spectrum disorders. New York: The Guildford Press; 2006. pp. 3-34.

[12] Elder J. In-home communication intervention training for parents of multiply handicapped children. Scholarly Inquiry for Nursing Practice. 1995;9:71-92.

[13] Flippin M, Crais ER. The need for more effective father involvement in early autism intervention. Journal of early intervention. 2011;33(1):24-50.

[14] Bendixen R, Elder J, Donaldson S, Kairella J, Valcante G, Ferdig RE. Perceived stress and family dynamics in fathers and mothers of children with autism following an in-home intervention. American Journal of Occupational Therapy. 2011.

[15] Smith L, Elder J. Siblings and family environments of persons with autism spectrum disorder: a review of the literature. Journal of child and adolescent psychiatric nursing: official publication of the Association of Child and Adolescent Psychiatric Nurses, Inc. 2010;23(3):189-95. Epub 2010/08/28.

[16] Lobato DJ, Kao BT. Integrated Sibling-Parent Group Intervention to Improve Sibling Knowledge and Adjustment to Chronic Illness and Disability. Journal of Pediatric Psychology. 2002;27(8):711-6.

[17] Fisman S, Wolf L, Ellison D, Freeman T. A longitudinal study of siblings of children with chronic disabilities. Canadian journal of psychiatry Revue canadienne de psychiatrie. 2000;45(4):369-75. Epub 2000/05/17.

[18] Hastings RP, Kovshoff P, Ward H, J. N, Espinosa F, Brown T, et al. Systems Analysis of Stress and Positive Perceptions in Mothers and Fathers of Pre-School Children with Autism. Journal of Autism and Developmental Disorders. 2005;35(5):635-44.

[19] Blacher J, Begum G. The Social and the Socializing Sibling: Positive Impact on Children with Autism. Exceptional Parent. 2009;39(5):56-7.

[20] Hodapp RM, Urbano RC. Adult siblings of individuals with Down syndrome versus with autism: findings from a large-scale US survey. Journal of Intellectual Disability Research. 2007;51(12):1018-29.

[21] Maynard AE, Martini MI. Learining in cultural context: Family, peers, and school. New York: Kluwer Academic/Plenum Publishers; 2005.

[22] Orsmond GI, Kuo HY, Seltzer MM. Father involvement with adolescents and adults with autism. 13th World Congress of the International Association for the Scientific Study of Intellectual Disabilities; Cape Town, South Africa2008.

[23] Baer D, Wolf M, Risley T. Some current dimensions of applied behavior analysis. Journal of Applied Behavior Analysis. 1968;1:92-7.

[24] Internet World Stats, (2010).

[25] Gentles JS, Lokker C, McKibbon AK. Health information technology to facilitate communication involving health care providers, caregivers, and pediatric patients: a scoping review. J Med Internet Res. 2010;12(2):e22.

[26] Fletcher PC, Markoulakis R, Bryden PJ. The costs of caring for a child with an autism spectrum disorder. Issues in comprehensive pediatric nursing. 2012;35(1):45-69. Epub 2012/01/19.

[27] NINDS, (2009).

[28] McConachie H, Diggle T. Parent implemented early intervention for young children with autism spectrum disorder: a systematic review. Journal of evaluation in clinical practice. 2007;13(1):120-9. Epub 2007/02/09.

[29] Lecavalier L, Leone S, Wiltz J. The impact of behaviour problems on caregiver stress in young people with autism spectrum disorders. Journal of Intellectual Disability Research. 2006;50(Pt 3):172-83. Epub 2006/01/25.

[30] Davis NO, Carter AS. Parenting stress in mothers and fathers of toddlers with autism spectrum disorders: associations with child characteristics. Journal of Autism and Developmental Disorders. 2008;38(7):1278-91. Epub 2008/02/02.

[31] Herring S, Gray K, Taffe J, Tonge B, Sweeney D, Einfeld S. Behaviour and emotional problems in toddlers with pervasive developmental disorders and developmental delay: associations with parental mental health and family functioning. Journal of Intellectual Disability Research. 2006;50(12):874-82.

[32] Hastings RP, Kovshoff H, Brown T, Ward NJ, Espinosa FD, Remington B. Coping strategies in mothers and fathers of preschool and school-age children with autism. Autism. 2005;9(4):377-91.

[33] Jones J, Passey J. Family Adaptation, Coping and Resources: Parents of Children with Developmental Disabilities and Behaviour Problems. Journal of Developmental Disabilities. 2005;11(1).

[34] Rao PA, Beidel DC. The Impact of Children with High-Functioning Autism on Parental Stress, Sibling Adjustment, and Family Functioning. Behavior Modification. 2009;33(4):437-51.

[35] Giarelli E, Souders M, Pinto-Martin J, Bloch J, Levy SE. Intervention pilot for parents of children with autistic spectrum disorder. Pediatric nursing. 2005;31(5):389-99. Epub 2005/11/22.

[36] Phetrasuwan S, Miles MS, Mesibov GB, Robinson C. Defining Autism Spectrum Disorders. Journal for Specialists in Pediatric Nursing. 2009;14(3):206-9.

[37] Sharpley C, Bitsika V, Efremidis B. Influence of gender, parental health, and perceived expertise of assistance upon stress, anxiety, and depression among parents of children with autism. Journal of Intellectual & Developmental Disability. 1997;22(1): 19-28.

[38] Beckman P. Comparison of mothers' and fathers' perceptions of the effect of young children with and without disabilities. American Journal on Mental Retardation. 1991;95:585-95.

[39] Bristol M, Gallagher J, Schopler E. Mothers and Fathers of Young Developmentally Disabled and Nondisabled Boys: Adaptation and Spousal Support. Developmental Psychology. 1988;24:441-51.

[40] Wolf L, Goldberg B. Autistic children grow up: An eight to twenty-four year follow-up study. Canadian Journal of Psychiatry. 1986(31):550-6.

[41] Trute B. Gender Differences in the Psychological Adjustment of Parents of Young, Developmentally Disabled Children. Journal of Child Psychology and Psychiatry. 1995;36(7):1225-42.

[42] Hastings RP, Johnson E. Stress in UK families conducting intensive home-based behavioral intervention for their young child with autism. Journal of Autism and Developmental Disorders. 2001;31(3):327-36. Epub 2001/08/24.

[43] Wong VC, Kwan QK. Randomized controlled trial for early intervention for autism: a pilot study of the Autism 1-2-3 Project. Journal of Autism and Developmental Disorders. 2010;40(6):677-88. Epub 2009/12/19.

[44] Myers SM, Johnson CP. Management of children with autism spectrum disorders. Pediatrics. 2007;120(5):1162-82. Epub 2007/10/31.

[45] Christison GW, Ivany K. Elimination diets in autism spectrum disorders: any wheat amidst the chaff? Journal of developmental and behavioral pediatrics : JDBP. 2006;27(2 Suppl):S162-71. Epub 2006/05/11.

[46] Group GDS. Gluten Free Casein Free Diet Success Stories. Gluten Free Casein Free Diet website: The GFCF Diet Support Group; 2012 [cited 2012 August 14]; Available from: http://www.gfcfdiet.com/successstories.htm.

[47] Knivsberg A, Reichelt K, Hoien T, Nodland M. A randomised, controlled study of dietary intervention in autistic syndromes. Nutrition Neuroscience. 2002;5(4):251-61.

[48] Whiteley P, Rodgers J, Savery D, Shattock P. A Gluten-Free Diet as an Intervention for Autism and Associated Spectrum Disorders: Preliminary Findings. Autism. 1999;3(1):45-65.

[49] Johnson C, Handen B, Zimmer M, Sacco K, Turner K. Effects of Gluten Free / Casein Free Diet in Young Children with Autism: A Pilot Study. Journal of Developmental and Physical Disabilities. 2011;23(3):213-25.

[50] Elder J, Shankar M, Shuster J, Theriaque D, Burns S, Sherrill L. The Gluten-Free, Casein-Free Diet In Autism: Results of A Preliminary Double Blind Clinical Trial. Journal of Autism and Developmental Disorders. 2006;36(3):413-20.

[51] Hyman JM, Zilli EA, Paley AM, Hasselmo ME. Working memory performance correlates with prefrontal-hippocampal theta interactions but not with prefrontal neuron firing rates. Frontiers in Integrative Neuroscience. 2010;4.

[52] Martin A, Cherubini A, Andres-Lacueva C, Paniagua M, Joseph J. Effects of fruits and vegetables on levels of vitamins E and C in the brain and their association with cognitive performance. The journal of nutrition, health & aging. 2002;6(6):392-404.

[53] Garcion E, Wion-Barbot N, Montero-Menei CN, Berger F, Wion D. New clues about vitamin D functions in the nervous system. Trends in Endocrinology & Metabolism. 2002;13(3):100-5.

[54] Mora JR, Iwata M, von Andrian UH. Vitamin effects on the immune system: vitamins A and D take centre stage. Nat Rev Immunol. 2008;8(9):685-98.

[55] Reynolds E. Vitamin B12, folic acid, and the nervous system. The Lancet Neurology. 2006;5(11):949-60.

[56] Golnik AEIM. Complementary Alternative Medicine for Children with Autism: A Physician Survey. Journal of Autism and Developmental Disorders. 2009;39(7): 996-1005.

[57] Amminger GP, Berger GE, Schäfer MR, Klier C, Friedrich MH, Feucht M. Omega-3 Fatty Acids Supplementation in Children with Autism: A Double-blind Randomized, Placebo-controlled Pilot Study. Biological Psychiatry. 2007;61(4):551-3.

[58] Brownstein J. Hyperbaric Autism Treatment Shows Possible Promise2009. Available from: http://abcnews.go.com/Health/AutismNews/story?id=7070353&page=1.

[59] Rossignol DA, Bradstreet JJ, Van Dyke K, Schneider C, Freedenfeld SH, O'Hara N, et al. Hyperbaric oxygen treatment in autism spectrum disorders. Medical gas research. 2012;2(1):16. Epub 2012/06/19.

[60] Offit P. Autism's False Prophets: Bad Science, Risky Medicine, and the Search for a Cure. New York, NY: Columbia University Press; 2008.

[61] Shute N. Alternative biomedical treatments for Autism: How good is the evidence? 2010:[3 p.]. Available from: http://www.scientificamerican.com/article.cfm?id=alternative-biomedical-treatments&page=2&WT.mc_id=SA_emailfriend.

[62] Unproven Treatments for Autism2010 August 13, 2012. Available from: http://www.webmd.com/a-to-z-guides/unproven-treatments-for-autism-topic-overview.

[63] Krishnaswami S, McPheeters ML, Veenstra-VanderWeele J. A Systematic Review of Secretin for Children With Autism Spectrum Disorders. Pediatrics. 2011;127(5):e1322-e5.

[64] Weber W, Newmark S. Complementary and alternative medical therapies for attention-deficit/hyperactivity disorder and autism. Pediatric clinics of North America. 2007;54(6):983-1006; xii. Epub 2007/12/07.

[65] Hoecker JL. Is chelation Therapy an effective autism treatment?2010. Available from: http://www.mayoclinic.com/health/autism-treatment/AN01488.

[66] Malone RP, Gratz SS, Mary Anne D, Hyman SB. Advances in Drug Treatments for Children and Adolescents with Autism and Other Pervasive Developmental Disorders. CNS Drugs. 2005;19(11):923-34.

[67] Rapin I. The Autistic-Spectrum Disorders. New England Journal of Medicine. 2002;347(5):302-3.

[68] West L, Waldrop J. Risperidone use in the treatment of behavioral symptoms in children with autism. Pediatric nursing. 2006;32(6):545-9. Epub 2007/01/30.

[69] King BH, Bostic JQ. An Update on Pharmacologic Treatments for Autism Spectrum Disorders. Child and Adolescent Psychiatric Clinics of North America. 2006;15(1):161-75.

[70] Dawson G, Rogers S, Munson J, Smith M, Winter J, Greenson J, et al. Randomized, Controlled Trial of an Intervention for Toddlers With Autism: The Early Start Denver Model. Pediatrics. 2010;125(1):e17-e23.

[71] Anderson SR, Romanczyk RG. Early Intervention for Young Children with Autism: Continuum-Based Behavioral Models. Research and Practice for Persons with Severe Disabilities. 1999;24(3):162-73.

[72] Wieder S, Greenspan SI. Climbing the symbolic ladder in the DIR model through floor time/interactive play. Autism. 2003;7(4):425-35. Epub 2003/12/18.

[73] Simpson RL. Evidence-Based Practices and Students With Autism Spectrum Disorders. Focus on Autism and Other Developmental Disabilities. 2005;20(3):140-9.

[74] Sundberg ML, Partington JW. Teaching language to children with autism or other developmental disabilities. Danville, CA: Behavior Analysts, Inc.; 1998.

[75] Combating Autism Reauthorization Act, Stat. S.1094 (2011).

[76] Committee IAC. Summary of Advances in Autism Spectrum Disorder Research: Calendar Year 20102010. Available from: http://iacc.hhs.gov/summary-advances/2010/.

[77] Smith T, Scahill L, Dawson G, Guthrie D, Lord C, Odom S, et al. Designing research studies on psychosocial interventions in autism. Journal of Autism and Developmental Disorders. 2007;37:354-66.

[78] Committee IAC. 2011 IACC Strategic Plan for Autism Spectrum Disorder Research. Department of Health and Human Services Interagency Autism Coordinating Committee website2011 [cited 2012 May 15].

Chapter 7

Collaboration Between Parents of Children with Autism Spectrum Disorders and Mental Health Professionals

Efrosini Kalyva

Additional information is available at the end of the chapter

1. Introduction

When mental health professionals and parents of children with autism spectrum disorders start working together, they bring into this relationship their own personal needs, concerns, priorities and responsibilities, which must be taken into consideration in order to create a mutually satisfactory and functional partnership. A partner is a person that one works with in order to achieve a common goal through shared decision-making and risk-taking. Some partnerships last for a short period of time and include casual encounters, while others last long and evolve through numerous official and unofficial encounters [1]. For a partnership model to work, all involved parties must understand how they feel about each other [2] and to recognize that family operates as a system. When parents and mental health professionals disagree, it is essential to resolve any conflict timely in order to avoid serious confrontations or even legal litigations [3].

Minuchin [4] was the first who introduced the theory of family systems and stated that individuals affect the context where they live and are in turn affected by it through a series of repeated interactions. So, whatever affects one family member affects the whole family in direct or indirect ways. Elman [5] describes families as the mobile that hangs over a baby's crib, with the pressure exerted on one end causing movement throughout. The relationships between family subsystems (spouses, parents and children, and siblings) determine the balance of the entire family [6] and interventions at any subsystem must aim to preserve this balance. For example, an intervention aiming at fostering the mother-child bond could affect the mother's relationship with her husband or her other children if the necessary actions are not taken. Family subsystems describe the interactions within the family context, whereas cohesion and adaptability describe the way in which family members interact.

Cohesion is inherent to the notions of engagement and disengagement. Some families with high levels of engagement do not have clear boundaries between the subsystems, are overly engaged in the therapeutic process and overprotective [4] and as a result do not allow the individual with autism spectrum disorders to develop a sense of autonomy. On the other hand, families with extremely low levels of engagement adopt rigid boundaries and do not interact with the child sufficiently. So, the child with autism spectrum disorders is left free, but without experiencing the necessary love and support. The degree to which a family adjusts to the diagnosis of autism spectrum disorders depends to a large extent on the pre-existing family cohesion and stability, while the disruption of family cohesion due to the birth of a child with autism spectrum disorders can lead to increased stress [7]. In order to deal with stress, families employ either internal coping strategies that include passive evaluation or active reframing or external coping strategies through social and spiritual support [8].

Adaptability refers to the family's ability to change its functioning when a stressful event occurs [9]. Family adaptability depends on the severity of autism spectrum disorders, as well as on the accumulation of the demands made on parents [10]. Rigid families do not change to face the stress, while chaotic families become unstable and face changes inconsistently. The families that do not manage to adapt successfully are at risk of becoming isolated and dysfunctional [11]. According to family systems theory the disruption of communication among family members is a sign of dysfunction of the whole system and not of a specific individual. Therefore, mental health professionals should aim at changing interaction patterns and not just individuals, without incriminating anyone. Many family members tend to blame the individual with autism spectrum disorders for the difficulties that they experience, but with the appropriate guidance they perceive that miscommunication is often to blame [12].

Most studies conducted with families of individuals with disabilities are based on the assumption that families are homogeneous [13], but there are many features that differentiate families between them. For example, unemployed parents of a child with autism spectrum disorders have access to different resources than high-income parents [1]. Moreover, single mothers of children with autism spectrum disorders experience heightened stress, since they lack the practical, financial and moral support of their partner [14]. Cultural and contextual factors can also affect the ways that families cope with disabilities. First generation Americans with Chinese origin are afraid that their children with autism spectrum disorders will be stigmatized if they use sign language or other alternative forms of communication [15]. Parental reactions to their child's disorders must be viewed and interpreted within the social, historical, and ecosystemic context of every family [16]. Parents initially experience a stage of shock [17], which is followed by a range of reactions that could eventually lead through consecutive reorganizations to adjustment to reality [18]. However, many parents regress to previous stages when they realize that their children with autism spectrum disorders face difficulties that will not disappear and that they need constant care. In order to support parents of children with autism spectrum disorders, mental health professionals must know the characteristics of the disorder and set realistic goals both for children with autism spectrum disorders and their families [19].

Many researchers have established that parents of children with disabilities and mental health professionals must cooperate in order to design and implement an effective therapeutic process [20-23]. Therefore, parental involvement in the planning of proper therapeutic intervention for children with autism spectrum disorders was the primary target of many programs since the beginning of the 1980s [24]. Parents have been treated as partners, consultants, advocates, and supporters by the mental health professionals who offer these services. Parents often seek to work together with mental health professionals as they try to help their children overcome the difficulties that they face [25-26]. So, empowering the cooperation between parents and mental health professionals has been a cornerstone for many contemporary care systems for individuals with disabilities [27]. In order to achieve this empowerment, it is important to increase parental autonomy and engagement in decision-making regarding the therapeutic goals [28].

It is expected that the cooperation between parents and mental health professionals will result to better services for the children with disabilities, since the knowledge and the experience that each person brings into this relationship are unique [29]. The problem is that many mental health professionals cannot treat parents as equal partners in this process [30]. Through their training, mental health professionals develop an area of expertise that places them almost automatically at the role of the expert. Sharing responsibility with parents, without having a clear hierarchy, creates a new structure that is opposite to the traditional nature of the relationship between parents and mental health professionals. However, the position and the authority of the mental health professionals have been challenged and transformed according to contemporary political and theoretical models, as can be seen below:

1.1. Professional as experts

This is the traditional cooperation model that is prominent in doctor-patient relationships, where the professionals use their position and their knowledge to decide what will happen. Parental participation is of secondary importance and compliance with the professionals' suggestions is self-evident. Parents are informed about the decisions that were taken without being allowed to express their opinions, feelings, needs, or wishes. Children are treated as the passive recipients of a therapy, while parents are thought not to have the time, the disposition, the skill or the knowledge to help their children. This relationship is very bureaucratic and rigid, because it disadvantages parents by making them dependent on the professional [31]. Moreover, when mental health professionals do not engage parents actively in their child's treatment there may be a disagreement between the therapeutic goals they set [31-32]. The exclusion of parents from the therapeutic process has been highly criticized since the beginning of the 1970s, since the relationship between parents and mental health professionals becomes impersonal and the sense of trust is lost [33]. Therefore, parents started gradually being involved in the therapeutic process [34] and a lot of emphasis was placed on this involvement [35]. It should be pointed out, that even though this kind of relationship is outdated, there are still mental health professionals who impose themselves on parents.

1.2. The transitional relationship

Mental health professionals started treating parents as co-therapists and realizing that the house can be used as a learning setting. They shared and transfered their skills to parents to help them become more able, more confident, and more skilled. Parents participate as «co-teachers» or «co-trainers» or «co-therapists» [18]. Mental health professionals have to adapt their methods in order to incorporate and to support their cooperation with parents. So, they have to discover ways to communicate with parents and to engage them in the therapeutic process. Parents who cooperate with mental health professionals become more able, more knowledgeable and more assertive [36]. The main drawback of this model is the underlying assumption that all parents have the motive (and are able) to use this professional knowledge to help their child. It ignores the differences that exist in parenting styles, family relationships, family resources, family values and cultural contexts. For example, some parents may not feel comfortable acting as «teachers» of their children [37]. Many interventions have focused solely on mothers and have left out fathers creating disruption to the family system. This relationship is not truly cooperative, since mental health professionals make the basic decisions and are still in control [31].

1.3. Parent as consumers

The consumer model [31] stated that parents should have new rights and be given part of the control. Parents are viewed as consumers, who have the right to choose the appropriate services and interventions for their children. It is the first time that mental health professionals recognize that parents possess specialized knowledge that they lack. Parents use their knowledge to decide what they want and what they need for their child. Mental health professionals guide parents to make more effective and appropriate decisions. Parents may choose not to attend some of the suggested services that they do not consider suitable. Decision-making is reached after mutual exchange of ideas and with mutual respect. The objective is to reach a mutual agreement on the treatment that the child will follow. This model can be quite effective in various intervention settings [38]. The cooperation is very important, since parents have a greater sense of control. The services that adopt this model must be very flexible to provide individualized support [39]. This model presupposes that parents are capable to express and to assert their needs and the needs of their children. However, some parents cannot prioritize their needs or assume the responsibility of making important decisions. The concept of parents as consumers who share resources may not be very realistic in a restrictive financial context that offers minimal services. In this case the consumers do not necessarily buy the best services and many parents cannot afford the increased financial demands of the most effective therapies. This model is similar to counseling that is offered to parents to help them resolve some personal issues.

1.4. The empowerment model

This model has added a social and systemic dimension to the consumer model [39], since parents have the right to choose the services that they will offer to their child and mental health professionals realize that family is a system and a social network. Every family comprises of interconnected social relations within the context of the family itself as well as within the wider social groups (extended family, friends, associates, cultural groups). The system and the network affect the ways in which the family members view the individual with disabilities. Given that each family has different advantages, parents have a unique adjustment method and mental health professionals need to understand and respect that. Mental health professionals should also help parents realize that they can monitor their child's progress and interfere when they identify a problem.

1.5. The negotiation model

Partners use negotiation to reach common decisions and to resolve any disagreements that may arise. Negotiation can lead either to a common decision or to disagreement. Disagreements can come up for various reasons, such as the priorities that are set by each interested party [40]. The negotiation model states that the ways that parents and mental health professionals view a situation or a problem, the options that they have to resolve it, and the extent to which they can face it, are affected by their roles – as well as the social, financial, and structural frames where they function. Therefore, according to this model, cooperation may be dysfunctional under the three following conditions:

1. Either parents or mental health professionals do not have the intention or the skill to work with each other and to enter a cooperative relationship. Personal experiences may decrease the likelihood to cooperate [1].

2. Either parents or mental health professionals make all decisions and are not willing to share responsibility [41].

3. If the interests, the views, the priorities and the values of parents and mental health professionals are contradictory, then their relationship may become competitive – even if they apply various conflict resolution strategies.

Some organizations are eager to engage parents in the therapeutic process not because they recognize parental rights but because of staff shortage or scarce financial resources [36]. Parents should be involved in decision-making regarding their children because mental health professionals need their cooperation to do their job properly. Parents will also have a chance to establish and generalize at home the skills that their children have mastered [38]. In order for parents – and especially mothers – to function as therapists, they must devote a lot of time to meeting with mental health professionals to receive the proper training [42]. Parents of children with disabilities need guidance and support to be effective in their role [43-45]; otherwise, they will loose their self-esteem and become ineffective [46].

For the negotiation model to work, it has to operate at five different levels: personal, interpersonal, organizational, institutional, and ideological [40]. The sense of cooperation encourages the productive combination of knowledge, skills, and sensitivities from both parents and mental health professionals. The six elements that characterize a cooperative relationship and differentiate it from other types of relationships are [47]: a) cooperation is optional; b) cooperation demands equity among the participants; c) cooperation is based on mutual goals; d) cooperation depends on shared responsibility and decision-making; e) people who cooperate share their resources; and f) people who cooperate are equally responsible for the outcome.

Within this model, mental health professionals should have a clearly defined relationship with parents that has four predetermined goals [48]: a) include parents in decision-making about their child; b) train parents to participate in decision-making about their child; c) help parents therapeutically to deal with some issues that stop them from functioning more effectively; and d) render parents capable to work effectively and meaningfully with their child through empowerment.

The negotiation model has many functioning aspects that facilitate the development of a cooperative relationship between parents and mental health professionals, since it is developmental and parents are not viewed as static agents. They are encouraged to develop and improve their skills to become more effective and to work on their personal issues. In order to meet with the demands of this new role, mental health professionals are often called to take on multiple roles and to become more flexible. They may need to act as mediators between the parents and other agents, as well as to fight for the rights of the parents and their children with disabilities – especially in times of financial and moral crisis.

1.6. How do parents feel about mental health professionals?

Individuals with autism spectrum disorders depend on their families for daily care and support that are essential for the successful implementation of any therapeutic intervention [49]. Therefore, it has been acknowledged that the needs of all the family members should be taken into consideration when designing an intervention [50]. Many highly recommended treatments for autism spectrum disorders [see 49, for more information] – such as Applied Behavioral Analysis [51], TEACCH [52] and Portage [53] – stress the importance of active parental participation in the therapeutic process, which results from the proper cooperation with mental health professionals. However, many parents claim that their participation in their children's therapy is minimal and restrained to six-monthly briefing meetings, while they are not informed that they could be more actively involved in the treatment process [54]. Parents must be treated as partners during the planning, implementation, and evaluation of the therapeutic approach and not just as observers or clients [55].

Many parents complain because they have to wait a long time to diagnose their children with autism spectrum disorders and they need to visit up to four different mental health professionals [54]. In a small scale study where parents of 25 children with autism spectrum disorders were interviewed, it was found that these parents have to take their children to different therapeutic settings, which is extremely time consuming. They work together with an average of six mental health professionals for a total of approximately 37 hours per week [56]. Since parents are often exposed to many diverse opinions and suggestions expressed by mental health professionals, they end up being confused and they need guidance to make the right choices and decisions [1]. Therefore, mental health professionals who work therapeutically with the parents of children with autism spectrum disorders should assume also a counseling role [57].

Parents need to be extremely persistent in order to ensure the services and the provisions that are necessary for their children with autism spectrum disorders [58-59]. Parents started questioning the power of mental health professionals when they formed groups to fight for their rights. An extreme example of disappointment with mental health professionals was the creation of a centre of counseling and support for the parents of children with special needs that was created by parents and to which mental health professionals had no access [2]. The parents who founded this centre stressed that it provided them with the opportunity to talk and to share their experiences – giving them, thus, the strength to deal with their daily problems.

Despite the fact that parents were overall satisfied with the mental health professionals they had worked with in the past, they generally felt that they had to fight in order to access the services that their children needed. They reported that many mental health professionals failed to communicate with each other and with the parents and this created a heightened sense of dissatisfaction. This was due to the fact that most children were monitored simultaneously by several mental health professionals who seemed to work in isolation without sharing information and common therapeutic goals. Furthermore, many parents supported that the services they received did not suffice to address their children's multiple and complex needs [3]. Moreover, some parents claim that they are tired of being accused for the problems that their children face [60] and that constant criticism does not help them become better and more effective parents. Paradoxically, although some mental health professionals view mothers as guilty, they involve them at the same time in their children's therapy [61].

Crawford and Simonoff [62] studied the attitudes of parents of children attending schools for emotional and behavioral disorders. Many parents believed that they felt stigmatized and isolated because of the problems that their children were facing. Although the stigma accompanying mental health problems or other disorders, such as autism spectrum disorders is well recognized, there is limited research on the topic. Parents feel lonely and without any support, but they hesitate to share their concerns with others, because they are afraid that they will be further stigmatized and held responsible for their children's problems. So, it is not surprising that parents were excited to meet with other parents who face similar problems and can offer them valuable support.

Parents of children with special needs are often dissatisfied with the way that mental health professionals behave and with the attitudes that they express. However, most relevant research has not studied the actual interaction between parents and mental health professionals, but they are based on parental anecdotal evidence that is usually negative [63-64]. If the behaviors that parents report are accurate, then they constitute a breach of the professional code of ethics [65] and should be seriously taken into consideration. On the other hand, many parents appreciate that mental health professionals try to understand the family dynamics and to address the individual needs of every family member [66] and there are also quite a few parents who mention that mental health professionals have done their best to help them and their children with autism spectrum disorders [54].

The mental health professionals who interact with children with autism spectrum disorders and their families come from different educational and theoretical backgrounds, as well as from different disciplines: specialized professionals (such as psychologists, speech therapists, and social workers), doctors, teachers or students. Despite the fact that the contribution of mental health professionals to the planning and effectiveness of the treatment has been widely acknowledged, more research is needed on identifying how they deal with practical problems that arise during the course of their interactions with parents of children with autism spectrum disorders. The role of mental health professionals and therapists has been approached primarily by the psychoanalytic perspective and most studies have focused only on the role of the teacher of children with autism spectrum disorders.

1.7. How do mental health professionals feel about parents?

The beliefs and the assumptions that mental health professionals hold regarding parental contribution to the appearance and maintenance of their children's problematic behaviors and disorders greatly affect their choice of offered therapies and the intervention strategies that they use when interacting with the specific families [67]. Even the term «professional» has been controversial, since some refer to the traditional definition of professional (e.g., doctors, lawyers, architects, university professors), while others use this term to refer to most working people (e.g., nurses, social workers, and teachers) [68]. The term «mental health professionals» is now used to include all the educated people who have received the appropriate training to work with individuals with disabilities. It is used to make the distinction between trained staff and volunteers, carers, or untrained helping staff who work with individuals with disabilities.

There are different sources of «socially acceptable» power for mental health professionals [69]: physical power, power to provide resources, power of profession, power of specialization and personal power. For many years now, the role of mental health professionals is predetermined to provide them with the power and the right to use their knowledge and their experience as they wish. They have resources at their disposal that they can share with children with disabilities and their families, as well as the specialized knowledge that they have acquired through their training. Mental health professionals are usually considered experts, since they are knowledgeable about an area or a topic. In case that some parents disagree or refuse to cooperate with mental health professionals, the latter have the right to stop providing their services. Mental health professionals can have considerable power and so many parents treat them with respect.

The attitudes and perceptions of mental health professionals regarding their relation with the parents of children with disabilities have not been adequately researched [70]. Smets [71] explored staff attitudes regarding parental involvement in a service for individuals with intellectual disabilities and found that staff believed that parents were either unaware or indifferent to their children's problems. Staff believed that parents were limited to the role of the external observer and they were happy to defer the responsibility of caring for their child to another person. However, the researcher stressed that the perception of the staff did not correspond to reality and to the actual needs of the families of the service users.

Some mental health professionals recognize the importance of working together with the parents, but they claim that they are not adequately trained or prepared to do so and they receive no support from their services [72-74]. To address this issue, it is important to better understand the skills and the behaviors that mental health professionals need in order to learn how to cooperate with parents [75-76]. Interpersonal skills, such as sensitivity towards the parents, clarity and respect are usually highly appreciated by parents who work together with mental health professionals in early intervention settings [77].

1.8. Cooperation between parents and mental health professionals

Cooperation is a term that was recently introduced to literature looking at the relationship between parents and mental health professionals, but is quite difficult to accomplish in practice given that it means different things to different people. Cooperation can be viewed as basic principle or theoretical viewpoint that is based on fundamental power exchange [78]. However, there are many organizational, geographical or financial obstacles in the cooperation between different groups of mental health professionals or between mental health professionals and service users – that is, parents of children with disabilities [79-81]. The potential cooperation between mental health professionals and parents is based mainly on the anticipation that there will be an increase in the number and quality of offered services. However, many mental health professionals feel threatened when they have to choose who will have access to each service, especially when the choices are limited [82].

The cooperation between parents and mental health professionals is not just desirable but also mandatory, since it is enforced by law in many countries [20, 83]. It has been widely accepted that a healthy cooperative relationship between parents and mental health professionals can lead to timely conflict resolution and benefit children with disabilities [84-85]. This cooperation is even more vital in early intervention programs, which are family-centered [86] and through parental empowerment [87] there is a greater sense of parental accomplishment [88].

Most relevant studies show that parents and mental health professionals are familiar with cooperative relationships through their interpersonal experiences [89-90]. Functional cooperative relationships are characterized by trust, respect, communication and shared vision that are essential to make decisions that will lead to increased communication [91], inclusion [92], and appropriate service provision for children with disabilities [93]. Some research also shows that teachers prefer to have a closer and more meaningful relationship with parents of children with disabilities [94]. The existence of supportive relationships among parents and mental health professionals is the most important determinant of a successful cooperative relationship [75].

Despite the existing legislations in some European countries and the wishes of both parents and mental health professionals, it is often extremely difficult to create successful and functional cooperative relationships [95-96]. For example, in the context of family-centered early intervention cooperation remains an utopia [86]. Although mental health professionals seem to favor cooperative relationships with parents, research shows that there is a big gap between theory and practice [97]. Relevant studies [98] that were conducted using either focus groups or interviews and questionnaires showed that the basic problem is that mental health professionals do not treat parents as equal partners and continue to maintain control. So, the failure to establish cooperative relationships is due to the fact that that there are no trusting and empowering relationships between parents and mental health professionals [11, 99].

This failure to create cooperative relationships could also be caused by the inadequate definition of cooperation [100] that hinders the quest for a common goal through functional interactions [101-103]. There are six factors that are essential for the establishment of a cooperative relationship between parents of children with disabilities and mental health professionals and form the basis of the partnership protocol that will be presented later on in the chapter [104]. These factors are:

a. communication: parents stressed that communication with mental health professionals must be honest, frequent and open, with no hidden agendas. Mental health professionals should inform parents also about unpleasant developments in the therapeutic process but without becoming rude or aggressive and without using jargon. Parents want to have access to information regarding other services that are available for their children. Communication should be a two-way process, with both parents and mental health professionals listening to each other without being critical. Mental health professionals seem to agree about the necessity of open and honest communication with the parents that can form the basis of a trusting relationship.

b. commitment: mental health professionals should not view what they do as a simple job that pays for their expenses and treat children with disabilities just as another client or case that is filed. They must value the individual and pay attention to the relationship with the whole family of the child with disabilities. It is noteworthy that some parents thought that mental health professionals should greet them if they meet somewhere in public as a sign of respect and professional commitment. Many mental health professionals recognized the importance of commitment and argued that they often have to deal with parents who do not want to be involved with the therapeutic process or get involved in decision-making regarding their child. However, this should not stop them from making the effort to work closely with the parents.

c. equity: mental health professionals must make conscious efforts to empower the families that they work with, recognizing the importance of parental knowledge instead of devaluing it. Parents should be encouraged to express their opinions and to be fully engaged in decision-making in the context of a constructive exchange of ideas. Attention is needed to keep the very thin line between empowering the parents and giving them too much independence that could jeopardize the therapeutic process.

d. skills: parents tend to admire the mental health professionals who make the difference by offering practical help both to them and to their children with disabilities and who are skilled and well trained. Mental health professionals should have high expectations from the children that they work with if they are going to try hard to make some progress and reach the goals that they have set. Parents appreciate the mental health professionals who have the strength and the will to be constantly updated about the new developments in their areas of expertise. Most mental health professionals referred to the skills that they expect from their colleagues but not from parents (this partly reflects their lack of trust in a cooperative relationship with the parents).

e.   trust: this term has three different meanings according to the context where it is used. It means reliability in the sense that mental health professionals should honor their promises any way they can. It is equal to security, in the sense that parents need to feel that their children with disabilities are safe both physically and emotionally when in the company of mental health professionals. The third dimension of trust is the discretion that mental health professionals should possess regarding the information that they share with colleagues about a child.

f.   respect: a sign of respect is that mental health professionals treat the child with disabilities as a human being and not as a label or a diagnosis, that they are polite, considerate, punctual, and up-to-date with recent developments in the field. Several parents mentioned that these simple rules of courtesy and proper behavior are often overlooked in daily encounters. Many mental health professionals admit that the lack of respect to parents can cause severe damage to the therapeutic relationship.

It is interesting to note that parents and mental health professionals seem to agree on what they think constitutes a desirable and proper cooperative relationship. They may differ in the importance that they place on each factor and in whether they identify it as essential or not for the success of the cooperation. Both sides recognize that for a cooperative relationship to work, both parents and mental health professionals should do their best keeping in mind the interests of the child with disabilities. This study [104] emphasizes that it is imperative to conduct further research to create guidelines to delineate the relationship between parents and mental health professionals, rendering it thus more satisfactory and more effective. This is the aim of the present study that aspires through the use of a partnership protocol to delineate the relationship between parents of children with autism spectrum disorders and mental health professionals – a need that was identified also by other researchers [16, 105].

Because of the heterogeneity of the symptoms and characteristics of autism spectrum disorders, the diagnosis usually does not provide useful suggestions for the appropriate treatment [106]. Successful therapeutic interventions develop when parents and mental health professionals work together as a coordinated and cooperative team [107]. In order to deal with the needs of children with autism spectrum disorders and their families the program COMPASS was created [54], which aims at the cooperation between staff and parents to design the most appropriate therapeutic intervention for each child. The greatest challenge that mental health professionals who work with the families of children with autism spectrum disorders have to face is to ensure that these children attend the therapeutic interventions that best suit their unique and complicated needs [108]. Parental attitudes and parental satisfaction are widely used as indications of the success of early intervention programs [109]. Since parents are the ones caring for their children with autism spectrum disorders, their views should be seriously taken into consideration by mental health professionals. Parental concerns and preferences can be used to improve offered services, while parental satisfaction can be translated into a measure of success of a therapeutic intervention [110].

The interaction between parents of children with autism spectrum disorders and mental health professionals is crucial in special needs education because of the high incidence of autism spectrum disorders in the school population and the lack of resources [111-112]. However, this interaction is often fragmentary and characterized by confusion, disappointment, and tension that result to low levels of cooperation and decreased quality of service provision to the child with autism spectrum disorders [111].

The relationship between parents of children with autism spectrum disorders and teachers is also worth exploring [113-114], especially given that many children with autism spectrum disorders have communication deficits and cannot express themselves and their needs [115-116]. Research so far suggests that trust is built almost exclusively on personal interactions, encounters, and exchanges. Every encounter between parents and teachers turns into an opportunity to expand and to strengthen the bonds of trust between the interested parties. Of course, if parents suspect that teachers are not worthy of their trust, then the bonds that are created are very fragile. Many parents seek to create a strong bond with their child's teachers, because they believe that this will benefit their child [11, 117]. In order to build up their trust, both parents and teachers should state clearly and openly their expectations from this relationship in an effort to minimize misunderstandings [118].

Mental health professionals often have to announce bad news to parents regarding their child's diagnosis and prognosis, which cause drastic and often negative changes in their lives [119-120]. Since parents have the unquestionable right to know the truth about their child's condition, the question is not whether the mental health professionals will share the news but how they will do it [120]. Many mental health professionals have been criticized for the abrupt way in which they communicate upsetting news to the parents [46] and the detrimental effects this can have on the parents is a matter of great concern [121]. However, if the briefing is done properly, then this can be extremely useful for them, since they will be able to understand their child's needs and design the appropriate treatment plan [122].

Despite the significant increase in knowledge about the causes and course of autism spectrum disorders [123] and the appreciation of the importance or early diagnosis [124], there have been no noteworthy changes in the information that parents receive in their first contact with mental health professionals. Some studies [125-126] have looked at the interaction between parents and mental health professionals during the dissemination of the assessment conclusions. It was found that mental health professionals are aware of the dilemma of delivering upsetting news and seek the active participation of the parents in a joint articulation of the problem. Some mental health professionals ask parents first to express their opinions about their child's problems and then they share the diagnosis to corroborate the parents' perspective [127]. Other mental health professionals present a series of related general and specific symptoms that lead to a specific diagnosis and then allow parents to state the final diagnosis [126]. Usually, mental health professionals try to bridge the gap between their views and parental views by modifying the diagnostic label, so as to comply with parental wishes and to balance the levels of optimism and pessimism [125].

Parental satisfaction is an important element for the evaluation of the services that are offered to children with disabilities and their families [128] and can be related to other family variables, such as stress or depression [129], increased empowerment [130] or increased school involvement [131]. Some qualitative studies have shown that parents who are not satisfied with their relationship with mental health professionals experience stress and do not feel welcome in the decision-making process regarding their children [59]. There are also some documented cases of parents who were so unsatisfied with the early intervention programs their children attended that they removed them from the program [132]. On the other hand, there are many qualitative studies of families that come from different cultural backgrounds and report that parents who are satisfied with the services provided to their children tend to engage more in their training [133].

Research on parental satisfaction asks parents to evaluate the quantity or the quality of the services that their children receive, as well as the nature of their relationship with mental health professionals [128, 131]. However, there is still a basic gap in identifying a widely accepted definition of parental satisfaction and which intervention model can be implemented to increase this satisfaction [77]. In a survey of satisfaction among 290 parents of children with autism spectrum disorders [134], it was found that most individualized educational plans were not developed in cooperation with mental health professionals, they did not reflect the views and the concerns of the family and they were not successfully coordinated by the many different people who run the services. In another similar study [108] it was reported that most of the 539 parents had difficulty finding about the available services and accessing them. They also claimed that they were not given any choice, that they had to fight for what they wanted and that ultimately the received services differed greatly from what they had originally asked for. Finally, more than half of the parents who participated in another study [135] complained that they were not fully informed about the available services or the structural changes that were taking place in different agencies and that they were unhappy with their cooperation with mental health professionals. All these problems seem to be even more prominent for the families of children with autism spectrum disorders who have to interact with various mental health professionals, such as pediatricians, psychologists, speech therapists and many others [136].

1.9. The present study

The concept of boundaries is inherent in human relations and cooperation and represents the rules and limitations that can create a sense of safety [137]. In strictly professional relationships the involved parties have a clearly defined role that they hesitate to deviate from. However, in many mental health services professionals may fulfill various practical, informative, and emotional needs of the individuals who use these services and their families [105]. Despite the fact that the codes of ethics of different professional bodies offer guidelines for the behaviors that protect mental health professionals against extreme cases of conflict of interest or client exploitation for own purposes, there are no guidelines for the delineation of daily interactions between mental health professionals and service users [138]. The code of ethics in special needs education does not address sufficiently the boundaries in relationships between mental health professionals and parents of children with disabilities [105] and this can hinder the establishment of a cooperative relationship between them [11]. So, it is imperative to create a form for the negotiation of the boundaries in daily interactions between parents and mental health professionals in order to make decisions about how, when and why the involved parties will interact [105]. This is how the partnership protocol that will be presented in this chapter was created on the basis of the codes of ethics of the British Psychological Society [139], the American Psychological Association [140], and the Health and Care Practitioners Council [141]. The aim of this study was to explore whether this partnership protocol could change the perceptions of parents of children with autism spectrum disorders and mental health professionals about their relationship. More specifically, it was hypothesized that parents of children with autism spectrum disorders would hold more positive attitudes about mental health professionals after the implementation of the partnership protocol. Mental health professionals would also express more positive attitudes towards the parents of autism spectrum disorders after the implementation of the partnership protocol.

2. Methods

2.1. Participants

The participants of this study were 40 mental health professionals working in the private sector with children with autism spectrum disorders and their families (18 men and 22 women): 5 psychiatrists, 10 speech therapists, 12 occupational therapists, 7 psychologists and 6 special educators. Their age ranged from 26 to 55 years old (mean age = 42 years and 2 months) and they have been working with children with disabilities from 3 to 30 years (mean years of professional experience = 17 years). The mean time that they have been working therapeutically with a child with autism spectrum disorders was 2 hours per week. Forty mothers and fathers of children with autism spectrum disorders from Northern Greece also took part in the study. There were 33 mothers and 7 fathers, aged 29 to 42 years old (mean age = 34 years and 7 months). Ten mothers were housewives, 17 were private employees, 9 were public employees, and 4 were self-employed. One quarter of the parents had one child, 24 had two children and 6 had three children. Most parents lived with their spouses, while 4 mothers were divorced and raised their children alone. All the parents had a child diagnosed with autism spectrum disorders from a public child psychiatric or child developmental clinic. The mean age of their child's diagnosis was 4 years and 8 months. Out of the 40 children with autism spectrum disorders there were 7 girls and 33 boys and their age ranged from 3.5 to 14 years old. Ten children attended special schools, 22 attended inclusion classes and the remaining 8 were in mainstream schools. The parents were in contact with more than 5 mental health professionals from the time they started seeking for a diagnosis and visited someone to help their children with autism spectrum disorders for an average of 5 years and 3.5 hours per week.

2.2. Measures

2.2.1. Partnership protocol

The partnership protocol (please see Appendix) is a document that aims to delineate the relationship between mental health professionals and the parents of children with autism spectrum disorders. It defines partnership as a «functional relationship characterized by a common goal, mutual respect and desire for negotiation». The protocol is two pages long in order to be handy and to offer condensed information in the 11 following areas: 1) cooperation between parents and professionals, 2) negotiation of boundaries in parent-professional relationship, 3) parental expectations/feelings/needs, 4) parental accuracy and reporting of knowledge, 5) parental understanding of their child's condition, 6) parental participation in decision-making, 7) parents as therapists, 8) parental briefing, 9) disclosure of information to parents or third parties, 10) family discord and 11) negotiation of parent-professional disagreement. The partnership protocol was piloted with five parents and seven mental health professionals.

2.2.2. Parent measures

The parents completed a brief questionnaire at baseline, which included the following information: gender, age, educational level, profession, number of children, age of child with autism spectrum disorders, gender of child with autism spectrum disorders, age of diagnosis of child with autism spectrum disorders, agency of diagnosis of the child with autism spectrum disorders, years of cooperation with mental health professionals, weekly contact frequency with mental health professionals and number of mental health professionals with whom they have cooperated so far. Then, parents were asked to define the relationship between parents and mental health professionals; to specify what they expect from cooperative mental health professionals; to mention the problems that they face from uncooperative mental health professionals; to describe what they do in case of disagreement with mental health professionals; to define negotiation and to judge if it is necessary for a successful therapeutic relationship; and to document the three advantages and the three disadvantages of their relationship with mental health professionals.

Parents were asked after the intervention to state whether the protocol was useful or not justifying their answers; whether any points needed further clarification; which were the most important points of the protocol; how often they used it; if it helped them define the nature of the relationship that they had with the mental health professionals; what happened in case of disagreement with mental health professionals; whether the protocol helped them resolve any disagreement with mental health professionals; and whether anything had changed in their relationship with mental health professionals.

In order to measure parental views about mental health professionals, the *Helping Behavior Checklist – (CBCL)* [142] was used, since it was based on the codes of ethics of six international organizations of mental health professionals. The first part, which was used in this study, consists of 16 statements that parents have to rate on a 4-point scale (where 1 = almost always true and 4 = almost never true), such as «the mental health professional clearly explained to me what I had to do to help my child», «the mental health professional did not involve me in any decision-making regarding my child's therapy» and «the mental health professional held me responsible for my child's problems». Scores are reversed in some items and the total score for the scale varies from 16 to 64. This questionnaire is highly correlated to parental satisfaction about their child's progress since they started working with the specific mental health professional. Test-retest reliability varies from 0.48 to 0.89 for a period of 2-3 weeks [142]. The Cronbach α of the scale for this study was high $\alpha = 0.89$ and deemed satisfactory.

2.2.3. Mental health professionals measures

The mental health professionals filled in a brief questionnaire at baseline with demographic information: age, gender, profession, years of professional experience, as well as weekly frequency of sessions with children with autism spectrum disorders. Then they were asked to define the relationship between parents and mental health professionals and what they expect from cooperative parents; to mention the problems that they face from uncooperative parents; to state whether their cooperation with parents is necessary for successful intervention; to describe what they do in case of disagreement with parents; to define the concept of negotiation and to judge if it is necessary for a successful therapeutic relationship; and to document the three advantages and the three disadvantages of their relationship with parents.

Mental health professionals were asked after the intervention to state whether the protocol was useful or not justifying their answers; whether any points needed further clarification; which were the most important points of the protocol; how often they used it; if it helped them define the nature of the relationship that they had with parents; what happened in case of disagreement with parents; whether the protocol helped them resolve any disagreement with parents; and whether anything had changed in their relationship with parents.

The views of mental health professionals about the parents of children with autism spectrum disorders they worked with were measured using *Providers' Beliefs About Parents Questionnaire (PBAP)* [143], which is based on some concerns that parents expressed about the attitudes or the behaviors of some mental health professionals who worked with their children with disabilities. It consists of 37 statements that mental health professionals have to rate on a 4-point scale (where 1 = completely disagree and 4 = completely agree). There are 5 subscales: a) «parental incrimination», which consists of nine statements, such as «the most common cause of severe emotional disorder in children is their parents' behavior» or «the most common cause of emotional problems in children is their parents' emotional inadequacy»; b) «necessity of informing parents», which consists of ten statements, such as «it is usually advisable to offer parent unlimited access to their child's files» or «all parents must be informed on how exactly a therapy is expected to help their child»; c) «recognition of parental status», which consists of seven statements, such as «parents of children in need of mental health services are usually emotionally involved to such an extent, that they do not accurately report their child's behavior» or «parents possess special knowledge that mental health professionals lack»; d) «attitudes towards drug use», which consists of six statements, such as «drugs usually help to deal with autism» or «the possible merit of drug therapy should be taken into consideration in most cases of autism»; and e) «providing guidance to parents», which consists of four statements, such as «it is not usually recommended to inform parents about what they can do exactly to help their child» or «it is therapeutically acceptable to brief parents directly about what they should do to help their child with autism». Scoring is reversed for some statements and the total score varies from 37 to 148. External validity ranges from 0.60 to 0.87 for each subscale [143] and test-retest reliability for the whole scale is 0.89 for a period of 2-3 weeks. Cronbach α for this study was very high for the whole scale ($\alpha = 0.93$) and is deemed extremely satisfactory.

2.3. Procedure

The researcher approached mental health professionals who were working privately with children with autism spectrum disorders in Northern Greece and briefed them about the study. She identified potential participants from the professional phone book and the lists of professional bodies in the area and then randomly pulled 100 papers with names from a container. She contacted them and 68 expressed an initial interest in the study, while 45 ended up agreeing to participate. The next step was to ask these mental health professionals to draw a list with the children with autism spectrum disorders they were working with at that time and the researcher randomly selected one family. The mental health professionals were given the task to brief the families and in case the parents expressed an interest the researcher met with them as well. There were some families who did not want to participate in the study, so another family was selected in their place until every mental health professional was matched to a family of a child with autism spectrum disorders. The parent from each family who participated was the one who was more in charge of the child's therapy and was in more frequent and direct contact with the mental health professional. This was deemed essential in order to follow the partnership protocol and to explore its effectiveness.

Before the beginning of the intervention the researcher informed the participants that they could withdraw at any time without penalty and that all the information that they provided would be confidential. Then, she gave out the baseline questionnaires that were filled out individually in the office of the mental health professionals and in the presence of the researcher. The next step was to present the partnership protocol to the participants in detail, to go through it with them and to answer any questions they might have. The intervention started when all participants reassured the researcher that they had fully understood the content of the partnership protocol and it lasted for six months. During this time the researcher called the participants monthly to check the progress of the data collection and to ask if there were any issues that needed to be addressed. Meanwhile, five parents discontinued the intervention at different points due to time restraints (one parent), health problems (two parents), or because they stopped taking their child to the particular mental health professional. So, the researcher asked the corresponding mental health professionals to stop using the protocol and the final number of participants was decreased to 40 parents of children with autism spectrum disorders and 40 mental health professionals.

Data collection was completed after a series of face-to-face meetings with every participant, who was asked after the intervention to fill in the same questionnaire as in baseline and to answer some additional questions about the protocol. The answers of the participants in the open-ended questions were explored with thematic analysis, which led to the categories that are presented. A second rater with experience with this type of analysis looked at approximately half of the data and the interrater reliability was extremely satisfactory (95.7%).

3. Results

Data analysis revealed that after the intervention parents of children with autism spectrum disorders were more satisfied with their cooperation with mental health professionals. Following the implementation of the partnership protocol mental health professionals tended to blame parents less for their children's problems, gave them more information about their children's situation and directions on how they should behave, while they also recognized more their parental status.

3.1. Parents of children with autism spectrum disorders

3.1.1. Baseline data

The characteristics of a satisfactory cooperative relationship between parents and mental health professionals according to parents were: honesty, mutual briefing, mutual trust and setting common goals. Parents believed that cooperative mental health professionals provide constant briefing on the child's progress (90%); implement the therapy with consistency (68%); are honest with parents (49%); recognize parental skills (40%); understand parental wishes and problems (35%); and really want to help (10%). Uncooperative mental health professionals, on the other hand, do not brief parents about their child's progress (88%); do not implement the therapy consistently (73%); are dishonest with parents (50%); do not understand parental wishes and aspirations (43%); withhold information related to the therapy (23%); and are not knowledgeable about autism spectrum disorders (20%).

The vast majority of the parents (88%) thought that it is essential to cooperate with mental health professionals in order for the therapy to succeed and approximately 75% reported that they should actively participate in their child's therapy. The rest of the parents considered that nothing can be done to alter the predetermined course that their children with autism spectrum disorders will follow. When a disagreement occurred with mental health professionals, most parents insisted and discussed with them when they believe that they were right, while they backed down when they were not certain. Parents defined negotiation as: clear expression of views from both sides; understanding with the child's progress as a common goal; arrangement of a time frame for the accomplishment of some results; and expression of realistic expectation from both parties. Indeed, almost 2/3 of parents (68%) reported that negotiation is essential for a successful therapeutic relationship. The advantages and the disadvantages that parents identified in their relationships with mental health professionals are presented in Tables 1 and 2 respectively.

	N	%
1. Encouragement about the child's progress	14	35
2. Genuine interest in the child and the family	10	25
3. Cooperation between parents and mental health professionals	7	17.5
4. Provision of practical advise to parents	5	12.5
5. Regular verbal communication with parents	3	7.5
6. Provision of support in all the areas of the child's development	1	2.5

Table 1. Advantages of Working with Mental Health Professionals According to the Parents of Children with Autism Spectrum Disorders

	N	%
1. Dishonesty about the child's progress	12	30
2. Lack of genuine interest in the child and the family	9	22.5
3. No understanding of parental needs	7	17.5
4. Inability to realize what is promised	5	12.5
5. Insensitivity to family's needs	4	10
6. Overcharging for the therapy	3	7.5

Table 2. Disadvantages of Working with Mental Health Professionals According to the Parents of Children with Autism Spectrum Disorders

3.1.2. Post-intervention data

Most parents (87%) stated that the partnership protocol was useful, because it provides a clear context for the relationships between parents and mental health professionals, it defines the roles of both parties, it promotes the positive cooperation that contributes to the child's progress and it familiarizes parents with their rights. The remaining 13% claimed that the protocol is not useful because it is binding and difficult to adhere to. Some parents said that the protocol should also clarify which qualifications mental health professionals should hold in order to work with children with autism spectrum disorders and what parents can do if mental health professionals do not follow the protocol.

The most important points of the partnership protocol were: ensured cooperation, honest relationships, understanding of parental limitations, parental participation in decision-making, and recognition of parental needs and emotions. Parents referred to the protocol every time that something changed in their child's therapy or a problem came up, as well as in case of disagreement with mental health professionals. The changes that parents observed in their relationship with mental health professionals after the implementation of the protocol were: parents and mental health professionals cooperated more effectively (32%); mental health professionals offered psychological support to parents (25%); mental health professionals took parental needs and expectations into account (19%); parents learned how to act as therapists for their children at home (13%); a time frame was set for the therapy (9%); and mental health professionals did not treat parents just as an income source (3%).

3.1.3. *The attitudes of parents of children with autism spectrum disorders towards mental health professionals*

Paired-samples t-test was use to compare differences in parental attitudes towards mental health professionals before and after the implementation of the partnership protocol. Before the intervention (M = 31.95, SD = 8.64) parents expressed statistically significant less positive attitudes towards mental health professionals ($t_{(1, 39)}$ = 107.25, $p < 0.001$, η^2 = 0.73) than after the intervention (M = 28.65, SD = 7.67).

3.2. Mental health professionals

3.2.1. *Baseline data*

The characteristics of a satisfactory cooperative relationship between parents and mental health professionals according to mental health professionals were: the exchange of ideas about the child, shared decision-making, mutual trust and respect, will to negotiate, and frequent contact. Mental health professionals believed that cooperative parents provide accurate information about their children (78%); follow their advise (68%); are honest about their child's condition (50%); are interested to learn more about their child (43%); do not have unreasonable expectations for their child's progress (42%); and actively participate in their child's treatment. Uncooperative parents, on the other hand, provide inaccurate information about their children (80%); question the mental health professional (60%); do not understand their child's condition (53%); do not keep certain agreements (45%); have irrational demands for their child's progress (38%); do not participate in their child's therapy (25%); and do not behave consistently (20%).

The vast majority of mental health professionals (93%) claimed that it is necessary to cooperate with parents for the success of the therapeutic intervention, since parents: possess valuable knowledge about their child that can be used in therapy, can complement the therapist's work and spend a lot of time with the child. In order to ensure parental cooperation, mental health professionals make parents feel more comfortable; brief them regularly about their child's progress; show sensitivity to the child's problems; express positive attitudes towards the child and the parents; promote parental beliefs that their child can improve with the proper therapy and support; take parental needs and wishes into account; engage parents in decision-making; gain parental trust; and try to specialize in autism spectrum disorders.

When mental health professionals disagree with parents, they tend usually to have an open and honest discussion with them, to engage them in decision-making, to be discrete, and to present their arguments. They may even resort to another mental health professional and in the end they make the final decisions if they cannot reach an agreement with the parents. Mental health professionals defined negotiation as exchange of ideas with the child's interest in mind, defining the boundaries of the cooperation, determining the expectations from

the therapy, setting mutual goals, discussing new possibilities, and compromising, if necessary. The advantages and the disadvantages that mental health professionals identified in
their relationships with parents are presented in Tables 3 and 4 respectively.

	N	%
1. Interest in their child's therapy	38	95
2. Willing to devote time to their child	35	88
3. Realistic expectations about their child's progress	27	68
4. Active participation in their child's therapy at home	22	55
5. Source of important information for the child	19	48
6. Willing to cooperate with mental health professionals	14	35
7. Trust mental health professionals	10	25
8. Wish a better future for their child	9	23
9. Encourage other family members to participate in therapy	6	15

Table 3. Advantages of Working with Parents of Children with Autism Spectrum Disorders According to Mental
Health Professionals

	N	%
1. No understanding of the child's condition	33	83
2. Emotional overload	30	75
3. Provision of inaccurate information	29	73
4. Refusal to engage actively in therapy	25	63
5. Exaggerated and unrealistic expectations	25	63
6. Unwillingness to cooperate	20	50
7. Lack of trust in mental health professionals	18	45
8. Feelings of parenting inadequacy	16	40
9. Insecurity for their child's future	15	38
10. Parental disagreements about their child	13	33
11. Rejection of the diagnosis of autism spectrum disorders	10	25
12. Experience of guilt over the child's condition	8	20
13. Crossing the boundaries (e.g., calling in the middle of the night)	6	15
14. Insisting on their views, even when they are wrong	10	4

Table 4. Disadvantages of Working with Parents of Children with Autism Spectrum Disorders According to Mental
Health Professionals

3.2.2. Post-intervention data

Most mental health professionals (80%) claimed that the partnership was useful, because it
sets the boundaries of the cooperation, it promotes negotiation, it emphasizes mutual respect, it clarifies the need for parental involvement in the therapeutic process and mental
health professionals have a reference point in case of disagreement. The remaining 20% stat-

ed that the protocol is not useful because it is binding and parents who are not educated cannot understand it. Some mental health professionals said that the protocol should clarify how much time mental health professionals should devote to parents, what happens when parents do not follow the protocol, and for which third parties mental health professionals should get the consent of the parents before they disclose information about their children.

The most important points of the partnership protocol were: the negotiation of the boundaries of the relationship between parents and mental health professionals, the clarification of the roles of both sides, and the emphasis placed on active parental involvement in their child's therapy. Mental health professionals referred to the protocol every time there was a disagreement with parents. The changes that mental health professionals observed in their relationship with parents after the implementation of the protocol were: parental expectations became more relevant to the child's condition (93%); parents realized that the whole family should be part of the therapy (80%); initial tensions were normalized (75%); parents felt that their expectations and emotions were taken into account (65%); parents were more committed to the therapy (58%); parents were more open to new suggestions and treatments for their child (35%); parents made less calls of hypothetical crises (23%).

3.2.3. The attitudes of mental health professionals towards parents of children with autism spectrum disorders

Analysis with MANOVA revealed that there was a statistically significant change in four out of the five subscales that measured the attitudes of mental health professionals towards the parents of children with autism spectrum disorders, even after being controlled for age, gender, and years of professional experience. More specifically, there were statistically significant changes in parental incrimination ($F_{(1, 39)}$ = 5.56, p < 0.05, η^2 = 0.12); necessity of informing parents ($F_{(1, 39)}$ = 5.03, p < 0.05, η^2 = 0.11); recognition of parental status ($F_{(1, 39)}$ = 4.83, p < 0.05, η^2 = 0.10); and providing guidance to parents ($F_{(1, 39)}$ = 5.35, p < 0.05, η^2 = 0.12). There was no statistically significant difference in the attitudes that mental health professionals expressed towards drug use before and after the intervention ($F_{(1, 39)}$ = 0.96, p > 0.05, η^2 = 002). Means and standard deviations are presented in Table 5.

	Baseline	Post-intervention	
	M (SD)	M (SD)	F
Parental incrimination	26.69 (3.54)	22.24 (3.44)	5.56*
Necessity of informing parents	14.15 (3.24)	17.93 (2.74)	5.03*
Recognition of parental status	14.06 (2.52)	19 (2.04)	4.83*
Attitudes towards drug use	6.11 (2.18)	8.41 (1.54)	0.96
Providing guidance to parents	3.25 (1.07)	8.17 (2.34)	5.35*

* $p < 0.05$

Table 5. Means and Standard Deviations of the Attitudes of Mental Health Professionals Towards Parents of Children with Autism Spectrum Disorders Before and After the Intervention

4. Discussion

The research hypotheses were confirmed, since both parents of children with autism spectrum disorders and mental health professionals expressed more positive attitudes about each other after the implementation of the partnership protocol. Most participants felt that the partnership protocol was particularly useful and they also identified some points that could be further clarified, while they also pointed out the exact nature of the changes that they have observed in their interactions.

4.1. The attitudes of parents of children with autism spectrum disorders towards mental health professionals

Most parents of children with autism spectrum disorders believed from the beginning that it was imperative to work together with mental health professionals in order to enhance their child's progress, while the rest believed that their child's progress was predetermined and there was nothing they could do to change that. Parents define a cooperative relationship as a relationship that is characterized by honesty, mutual briefing, mutual trust, and setting common goals [27]. The information that parents receive from mental health professionals is more important to them than sympathy or psychological support [144-145].

Parents describe cooperative mental health professionals as constant providers of update regarding their child's progress, consistent, honest, understanding, willing to help, and aware that parents possess certain skills. So, the parents in this study have identified essentially the defining characteristics of cooperative relationships [77]. Parents cannot cooperate with mental health professionals who do not brief them, are inconsistent and insincere, ignore them, withhold information and are not well trained – in agreement with other research [24, 28, 117].

The implementation of the partnership protocol helped the parents of children with autism spectrum disorders to redefine their cooperative relationship with mental health professionals. They learned to function as therapists at home, facilitating thus the therapeutic process [25-26]. They received emotional support from mental health professionals and they set a time frame for some therapeutic goals, which could help them feel less stressed [146]. Most parents reported that after the intervention mental health professionals treated them as more equals, briefed them about their child's progress, engaged them more actively in the therapeutic process, and took their feelings and opinions into consideration. This change may be due to the fact that a trusting relationship was created through the protocol, which helped the parents express themselves more freely and become more assertive. Trust is imperative for the creation of a constructive cooperative relationship between mental health professionals and parents of children with disabilities [104]. Many parents actively seek to create this bond of trust, since they feel that it will benefit their child [11, 117].

An additional change that was reported by the parents of children with autism spectrum disorders was that the mental health professionals started briefing them more about the ways in which the proposed therapy will help their child and encouraged them to get actively involved in decision-making regarding their child's treatment. Active participation in their child's therapy can help parents develop a sense of efficacy and personal control that can help them become even more effective parents [87] and less stressed and concerned [147]. When parents feel heard and respected, then they can cooperate better with mental health professionals to do what is best for their child and this is something that mental health professionals should aim at [66].

4.2. The attitudes of mental health professionals towards parents of children with autism spectrum disorders

Mental health professionals tended to incriminate parents of children with autism spectrum disorders less after the implementation of the protocol. This is very important, since it affects greatly the choice of suggested therapies and strategies that mental health professionals employ when interacting with the parents of children with autism spectrum disorders [67]. Since parents of children with autism spectrum disorders have been repeatedly blamed for the problems that their children face [148], the partnership protocol encourages the creation of a relationship that frees parents from guilt and treats them as equal partners. After the implementation of the partnership protocol, mental health professionals realized that it is essential to inform parents about their child's condition and the course of the therapy. The needs of all family members are taken into consideration [50] and, therefore, frictions are decreased [3, 11, 99]. So, it is possible to create a strong cooperative relationship that can benefit both parties [40, 47], while children with autism spectrum disorders can also benefit from parental empowerment [149].

The mental health professionals who adopted the protocol said that they recognized more the validity of parental knowledge and information regarding their child with autism spectrum disorders. This change is very positive, since parents of children with autism spectrum disorders know a lot of things about their children that are useful when planning the appropriate intervention [61]. The acknowledgement of the usefulness of parental knowledge by mental health professionals is essential to the cooperative process [60] and is, thus, emphasized in the partnership protocol.

Moreover, mental health professionals understood that they need to provide more clear and more detailed information to parents about the management and upbringing of their children with autism spectrum disorders. The partnership protocol stressed that parents can be trained to satisfy the needs that arise from their parenting role and this is instrumental for various therapeutic approaches [16]. Parents who receive specific guidance on how to deal with challenging and unwanted behaviors believe that they can control them better [150] and so they feel less stressed [146]. However, it is worth pointing out that some parents cannot or do not want to fulfill their instructional role [151] and this is something that mental health professionals should respect.

The statistical analysis revealed that the perceptions that mental health professionals hold about the parents of children with autism spectrum disorders were not affected by their age, gender, or years of professional experience. Therefore, it is likely that they are affected by their training and by the «social representations» that they hold about parents of children with autism spectrum disorders [152], as well as by cultural and social factors [18].

Almost all the mental health professionals believed that their cooperation with the parents of children with autism spectrum disorders was essential to the successful course of the therapy [86, 128], since they bring their own knowledge and experience into the therapeutic process [29]. Therefore, they claimed that in order to ensure this cooperation they try to earn parental trust and to make them feel comfortable, while taking into account their needs and wishes. By briefing parents about their child's progress, they engage them more actively in decision-making regarding the treatment course [93]. However, it is worth mentioning that at the beginning of the study parents complained that mental health professionals do not try enough to cooperate with them. This could be due to a wider communication problem that has been documented also in other studies, since good intentions alone are not enough to establish cooperation [86, 94]. Finally, mental health professionals claimed that they tried to increase their knowledge through training in order to be able to better deal with the problems of children with autism spectrum disorders. This needs to be done if mental health professionals are to design an intervention that is based on the child's needs and skills and is more likely to be successful [49].

Mental health professionals define cooperation as a relationship that is characterized by exchange of views about the child, shared decision-making, mutual trust and respect, desire to resolve disagreement, frequent contact and discussion on equal terms (there is no expert) [15, 59, 89, 93]. This definition that they provided includes some of the key characteristics of the negotiation model [40].

Parents should provide accurate information about their child that is essential for the establishment of a cooperative relationship with mental health professionals [77]. Otherwise, mental health professionals have to waste a lot of valuable time and resources to find out what they need to design an effective intervention [1]. Parents who are unaware of their child's actual condition may place irrational demands on both their child and mental health professionals and fail to keep agreements and deadlines, jeopardizing their child's progress [111]. Finally, there are some parents who question the training of mental health professionals and their suitability to work with their child, but may continue to cooperate because they have no other options or because they believe they can motivate the mental health professional [11, 99].

Mental health professionals noted that after the implementation of the partnership protocol parents started to have more realistic expectations that made them realize the importance of engaging the whole family in the therapeutic process [54]. Parents understood that they have to follow the advice of mental health professionals to help their children and became more open to new treatment suggestions [104]. These behaviors are indicative of greater trust for the mental health professionals, who need initially to recognize the shock that parents experience [17] and to help them reach the stage of full acceptance [16]. Parents also seemed to have responded positively to the efforts made by mental health professionals to take their feelings and views into account when designing the intervention [75]. Finally, mental health professionals reported that the parents were better able to judge when they needed to communicate in order to resolve an actual crisis, probably as a result of their active therapeutic engagement [98].

4.3. Evaluation of the partnership protocol

Most parents of children with autism spectrum disorders and mental health professionals who used the partnership protocol said that it was useful, because: a) it clarifies the relationship between the two parties; b) it defines the roles of both parties; c) it promotes effective cooperation; d) it advances negotiation; and e) it values mutual respect. All these elements were rated by many studies [28, 101, 103] as essential for the creation of a functional and effective cooperative relationship among parents and mental health professionals. It is extremely important to point out that both parents and mental health professionals recognize similar benefits from the implementation of the protocol, corroborating the finding that the needs of parents and mental health professionals are closer that one would think, but they need to be clearly defined in order to be satisfied [100].

The parents of children with autism spectrum disorders reported that the partnership protocol informs them of their rights and helps them fight for provisions and services. Parental participation is instrumental in reassuring the existence of options for adults with autism spectrum disorders [153]. Parents become empowered [39, 86] and thus able to negotiate with mental health professionals [40]. Mental health professionals said that they could use this protocol to resolve conflicts or disagreements with parents. This is important, since some mental health professionals do not know how to resolve interpersonal conflicts [3] and they become increasingly stressed [147].

The four parents who thought that the partnership protocol is not useful justified their opinion by saying that it is binding and difficult to adhere to. It is a fact that the implementation of a protocol or any form of agreement requires commitment from all involved parties. Therefore, it is likely that some parents of children with autism spectrum disorders are exhausted from the constant care of a child with multiple and complex needs and do not possess the required strength to enter this process [146]. Moreover, it is plausible that some parents prefer to hold a more distant role from the therapeutic process [54]. The eight mental health professionals who considered the partnership protocol not to be that useful thought as well that it is binding and that parents who are not educated cannot understand it. It seems that they do not want to be committed to a predetermined cooperative relationship with the parents because they have adopted the expert model. Even if some parents are not educated or able to understand some points, it is the role of mental health professionals to explain everything to them in simple and understandable language [56].

Approximately 20% of the parents of children with autism spectrum disorders identified two things that needed further clarification in the partnership protocol: a) which qualifications mental health professionals should hold in order to work with children with autism spectrum disorders and b) what parents can do if mental health professionals do not follow the protocol. The first point partly reflects the insecurity that results from insufficient briefing regarding the options that parents have to choose the suitable mental health professional after the diagnosis [55]. They could also result from limited options due to place of residence or financial restraints [99]. The second clarification is indicative of feelings of inferiority or intimidation. This partnership protocol has no legal power and it is not a contract with legal ratifications. The whole point of the protocol is to introduce parents to the concept that they can discuss any conflict or disagreement with mental health professionals on equal terms.

Mental health professionals also wanted to know what will happen in case that parents of children with autism spectrum disorders do not follow the protocol. This is something that should be discussed and agreed upon from the beginning between the two parties. Most disagreements are peacefully resolved, while very few have ended up in court [3]. Moreover, it is important that some mental health professionals realize that some parents will not want to cooperate with them [76]. The second question was how much time mental health professionals should spend with parents of children with autism spectrum disorders and this is again to be negotiated between them from the beginning.

The most important positive outcomes of the partnership protocol are: ensured cooperation, honest relationships, understanding of parental limitations, parental participation in decision-making, and recognition of parental needs and emotions. It seems that what parents really need is to feel like equal partners in the therapeutic process and this is something that the partnership protocol offers. Parents who are involved in decision-making about their child and are supported by mental health professionals feel happier [2, 33, 154]. The most important positive outcomes of the partnership protocol are: the negotiation of the boundaries of the relationship between parents and mental health professionals, the clarification of the roles of both sides, and the emphasis placed on active parental involvement in their child's therapy. Mental health professionals need to define their relationships with parents as much as parents do [28, 77-78] and they use the protocol to do so.

4.4. Limitations

The aim of this study was to create a partnership protocol to delineate the relationship between parents of children with autism spectrum disorders and mental health professionals with the ultimate goal to improve the child's condition [84]. The need for this protocol derived from personal experience and from meticulous literature search [16, 105]. Although the findings were positive and encouraging, there are some limitations that should be taken into consideration:

1.   The mental health professionals were working in the private sector and so they might be more willing to follow the protocol in order to keep their clients – things could be different if they worked in a public setting.

2.   The mental health professionals who agreed to participate in the study might have been the ones who work better with parents, and the parents who participated might have been the ones who were happy with mental health professionals to begin with. However, analysis showed that all the participants identified some problems at baseline.

3.   Some confounding variables, such as the training of mental health professionals or the educational level of the parents were not taken into consideration when analyzing the findings. For example, it was found that single mothers of children with autism spectrum disorders experience more stress than married mothers [14].

4. Despite the fact that the participants were reassured that data would be kept confidential, they might be skeptical about expressing very negative attitudes [155].

5. There was no official follow-up, although the researcher had informal contacts with the participants and was informed that many of them continued to follow the partnership protocol after the six-month period.

6. There are many other factors that could have affected the collaboration between parents of children with autism spectrum disorders and mental health professionals that are related to external factors (e.g., financial crisis), internal factors (e.g., depressive mood) or child-specific factors (e.g., severity of the autism spectrum disorders) that were not examined in the present study and could inform further research.

4.5. Practical implementation and future research

This research confirmed the findings of previous studies [77, 104, 147] that the relationship between parents of children with autism spectrum disorders and mental health professionals is quite challenging. However, the aim was not just to identify the existing problems, but to propose also some possible solutions. It seems that the implementation of the partnership protocol had a positive effect on the delineation of the relationship of the involved parties and helped them overcome some the existing obstacles by becoming more cooperative and willing to negotiate for the child's benefit.

As mentioned in the introduction, mental health professionals and parents of children with disabilities hold their personal beliefs regarding the kind of relationship that they should have. The partnership protocol helped them understand their rights and obligations, since they might hesitate to discuss them openly. There are many mental health professionals who do not know how to set limits to their relationships with parents and many parents who do not know how to express their opinions or their questions regarding their child to mental health professionals. Therefore, the partnership protocol may be suggested by mental health professionals as a means to negotiate their relationship with parents, while it serves also as an opportunity to discuss further and to resolve any conflicts. However, it should be stressed that the partnership protocol is not a legally binding document and so parents and mental health professionals should follow it because they believe in its value. It can be implemented in any therapeutic framework, where it is essential for parents of children with disabilities and mental health professionals to work together. It could also be used to train mental health professionals who will work with children and adolescents with disabilities and their families [156].

This is the first study in Greece, and worldwide, that introduced the use of a partnership protocol to resolve possible conflicts that arise between mental health professionals and parents of children with autism spectrum disorders. Therefore, future studies should be conducted with parents of children with other disabilities, as well as with parents of children with chronic illnesses and with other mental health professionals, such as doctors, nurses, or teachers.

5. Conclusion

This study confirmed the findings of previous international research regarding the problematic relationships between mental health professionals and the parents of children with disabilities. It was found that Greek mental health professionals are troubled by the parents' demands and their unwillingness to actively engage in their child's treatment. Greek parents of children with autism spectrum disorders claim that mental health professionals are not interested in involving them in decision-making regarding their child's therapy. Similar complaints have been expressed in other studies that have explored the relationship between mental health professionals and parents of children with autism spectrum disorders [77, 104, 147].

Despite the fact that the difficulties that were documented in this study have been identified a long time ago and in several contexts, there has been no published coordinated effort to resolve them. This partnership protocol was based on the codes of ethics of international organizations of mental health professionals, it is written in simple language and it was considered to be useful by most participants. The implementation of the partnership protocol helped mental health professionals and parents of children with autism spectrum disorders to define their interpersonal relationship and to overcome many of the difficulties and the problems that they had identified at the beginning of their cooperation. They started to communicate more honestly, to respect each other more and to resolve their conflicts more effectively. Even though these findings are encouraging, more longitudinal studies with varied participants are needed to explore further the effectiveness of the partnership protocol.

Acknowledgement

I would like to thank all the participants and Dr Angeliki Gena who was the primary supervisor of my second PhD that is the basis of this research. I extend my gratitude also to my family and especially my husband and colleague Vlastaris Tsakiris for his constant support throughout this lengthy process.

Appendix

Parent-Professional Partnership Protocol

When professionals and parents of children with autism come together for the first time, they bring with them their own worries, concerns, priorities, and responsibilities, which must be woven together into a relationship that could be characterized as a partnership. The roles of the parent and the professional impose certain rights and duties, obligations and anticipated behaviours, as well as expectations. It is extremely difficult to define the exact nature of this partnership, since every parent and every family has its own idiosyncrasies and each professional possesses unique characteristics and ways of working and relating. The aim of the present document is to provide some guidelines that could be adopted and implemented by both interested parties in an attempt to define their partnership and it is based on the principles of the negotiating model. The negotiating model defines partnership as "a working relationship that is characterized by a shared sense of purpose, mutual respect and the willingness to negotiate".

Cooperation between parents and professionals

Professionals need parental cooperation in order to be able to do their job effectively. Parents should recognize that professionals have specialist knowledge and abilities, but they cannot substitute the role of the caregiver. Since both parents and professionals are interested in the child's progress, they need to cooperate to achieve the best results.

Negotiation of boundaries in parent-professional relationship

Parents and professionals should clarify and negotiate the nature and the limits of their partnership. It would be advisable to make a contract that is not formal or legally binding. It just sets out mutual expectations and intended behaviours. Depending on the situation it may be appropriate to put this in writing and each party should retain their own copy. It is advisable to repeat this process at later stages according to the progress of the child. Parents should refrain from contacting the professional on a regular basis about things that do not concern the child with autism and professionals should be punctual and fulfil their obligations towards the family and the child.

Parental expectations/feelings/needs

Professionals should identify and evaluate the needs of the family, which cannot be separated from the needs of the child. The child has a relationship with all the other family members and the relationships within the family have an interactive effect with each other. Parents should verbalise and express their urging needs to professionals so that a solution can be sought. These expectations, feelings, and needs should be incorporated into the treatment when the professional believes that is plausible and suitable.

Parental accuracy and reporting of knowledge

Parents possess a unique and special knowledge and understanding about their child that is valuable for the design of a better intervention. The home is the best available place to consolidate the knowledge that the child acquires and it can also offer multiple opportunities for learning. Parents should be honest with professionals and try to overcome the difficulty they may experience to talk publicly about the condition and the difficulties of their child. If the professional is misled or told half the truth, it is very likely that the suggested treatment will not be the appropriate one.

Parental understanding of their child's condition

Professionals should use simple language when talking to parents, since they do not have expert knowledge that allows them to familiarise themselves with terms used among professionals. Parents should also express their queries and seek to clarify any misconceptions or worries they might have. If parents believe that they are not being listened to, they should make sure that the attitude of the professional changes. Professionals must not focus on the child alone, but they should advise parents on how to care for their child with autism. Even if parents have other children, they may need some practical assistance and tips on how to overcome some of the issues that arise due to the difficulties faced by their child. It is the parents' responsibility to inform professionals on the areas where they believe they need more help and support.

Parental participation in decision-making

Professionals should allow parents to be more involved in activities and decisions regarding the education and care of their child. For example, professionals should not make drastic changes in the treatment that they follow before consulting with the parents. This is a good way to ensure cooperation and to minimise conflicts in parent-professional relationship. Parents will be able to make an informed choice regarding the future of their own child. Therefore, a common purpose or shared concern or mutual interest should be established in order for the relationship between the interested parties to be productive. Both parents and professionals should be involved in brainstorming regarding potential ideas, plans, or actions that could enhance the development of the child. Parents should make an effort to follow and understand the progress of their child in order to be able to make a decision. This could include reading books, notes, or reports regarding the condition of their child and the treatment that is implemented.

Parents as therapists

Professionals may train parents to use some behavioral techniques that will allow them to teach their child, complementing thus and supporting the work of professionals. If parents feel confident enough, they may want to assume an active role in furthering their child's learning. However, professionals should be aware that parents may not have enough time to be actively involved in the education of their child if they have a full-time job or other children to look after. Therefore, at the beginning of the partnership professionals and parents should reach an agreement on the amount of time that parents can spend with their child on a weekly basis. Professionals should encourage each member of the family to contribute to the treatment of the child with autism, which may need special assistance to participate in family outings and activities. This can be achieved by encouraging parents to communicate with each other and express openly their concerns and needs.

Parental briefing

Professionals should inform parents from the beginning about the cost of the treatment, seek their consent when contemplating the acquisition of new material, and brief them about the progress of their child, even if the news are not particularly encouraging or reassuring. It would be a good idea for professionals to keep notes of the meeting with the parents, so that they can refer to them in the future and keep track of the progress of their child.

Disclosure of information to parents or third parties

Professionals could verbally inform parents about the progress of their child but access to records may be prohibited due to legal issues related to their confidentiality – professionals are called to make individual decisions according to each situation. Parents who advocate their right to have access to the records should be equally responsible in their own record keeping. Professionals should inform parents of any other professionals with whom they discuss the case of their child and elicit their consent before doing so.

Family discord

In case of disagreement between the parents regarding the treatment of their child, professionals should stay neutral and avoid making alliances with one parent or colluding consistently with one parent's preferences. If professionals believe that there are many pressing issues among the family members, they should encourage them to see a counsellor. Parents should realize that professionals working with their child may not have the necessary knowledge and training to deal with these issues.

Negotiation of parent-professional disagreement

When a disagreement arises, both parents and professionals should try to resolve it. They must express their opinions and feelings openly, keeping in mind that they have the child's best interest in mind. If it is impossible to resolve the disagreement, it might be advisable to discontinue the partnership.

Author details

Efrosini Kalyva

Address all correspondence to: kalyva@city.academic.gr

Psychology Department, The International Faculty of the University of Sheffield, CITY College, Thessaloniki, Greece

References

[1] Seligman M, Darling RB. Ordinary Families, Special Children: A Systems Approach to Childhood Disability. 2nd ed. New York: The Guilford Press; 1997.

[2] Swain J, Walker C. Parent-Professional Power Relations: Parents' and Professionals' Perspectives. Disability and Society 2003;18(4) 547-560.

[3] Feinberg F, Beyer J, Moses P. Beyond Mediation: Strategies for Appropriate Early Dispute Resolution in Special Education. Unpublished manuscript. National Center on Alternative Dispute Resolution (CADRE): Eugene, OR; 2002.

[4] Minuchin S. Families and Family Therapy. Cambridge, MA: Harvard University Press; 1974.

[5] Elman NS. Family Therapy. In Seligman M. (ed.) The Family with a Handicapped Child. 2nd ed. Boston: Allyn & Bacon; 1991, p369-406.

[6] Turnbull AP, Summers JA, Brotherson MJ. Family Life Cycle: Theoretical and Empirical Implications and Future Directions for Families with Mentally Retarded Members. In Sowers J. (ed.) Making our Way: Promoting Self-Competence among Children and Youth with Disabilities. Baltimore: Brookes; 1986, p45-66.

[7] Weiss S. Stressors Experienced by Family Caregivers of Children with Pervasive Developmental Disorders. Child Psychiatry and Human Development 1991;21(2) 203-216.

[8] Siklos S, Kerns KA. Assessing Needs for Social Support in Parents of Children with Autism and Down Syndrome. Journal of Autism and Developmental Disorders 2006;36(7) 921-933.

[9] Grissom M. "From their own perspective": An Ethnographic Study of Families with Children with Autism. Dissertations Abstracts International: The Sciences and Engineering. 2005;65 3745.

[10] Pakenham KI, Samios C, Sofronoff K. Adjustment in Mothers of Children with Asperger Syndrome: An Application of the ABCX Model of Family Adjustment. Autism 2005;9(2) 191-212.

[11] Turnbull AP, Turnbull HR. Families, Professionals, and Exceptionality: Collaborating for Empowerment. 4th ed. Columbus, OH: Merrill; 2001.

[12] Turnbull AP, Patterson JM, Behr SK, Murphy DL, Maquis JG, Blue-Banning MJ. Cognitive Coping, Families, and Disability. Baltimore: Brookes; 1993.

[13] Turnbull AP, Turnbull HR. Families, Professionals and Exceptionality: A Special Partnership. 3rd ed.Upper Saddle River: Merrill; 1997.

[14] Bromley J, Hare D, Davison K, Emerson E. Mothers Supporting a Child with Autistic Spectrum Disorders: Social Support, Mental Health Status and Satisfaction with Services. Autism 2004;8(3) 409-423.

[15] Parette P, Chuang SJL, Huer MB. First Generation Chinese American Families' Attitudes Regarding Disabilities and Educational Interventions. Focus on Autism and Other Developmental Disabilities 2004;19(1) 114-123.

[16] Gena A. Family and Child with Autism: Parental Reactions and Adjustment. In Gena A, Kalogeropoulou E, Mavropoulou S, Nikolaou A, Notas S, Papageorgiou V. (eds.) The Autism Spectrum: Cooperation between family and professionals. Trikala: The Association of Parents and Friends of Children with Autism; 2006, p45-88.

[17] Gena A. Autism and Pervasive Developmental Disorders. Athens: Author; 2002.

[18] King Gerlach E. Part 1. The Beginning: How Parents Move Forward and Make
      Choices after Diagnosis. Exceptional Parent Magazine, New York: www.discov-
      ery.org-www.thecenterfordiscovery.org; 2002.

[19] Rolland JS. Mastering Family Challenges in Series Illness & Disability. In Walsh F.
      (ed.) Normal Family Processes. 2nd ed. New York: Guildford Press; 1993, p444-473.

[20] Adelman H, Taylor L. Addressing Barriers to Learning: Beyond School-Linked Serv-
      ices and Full Service Schools. American Journal of Orthopsychiatry 1997a; 67(3)
      408-421.

[21] Adelman HS, Taylor L. Toward a Scale-up Model for Replicating New Approaches
      to Schooling. Journal of Educational Psychology Consultation 1997b;5(2)197-230.

[22] Children's Aid Society. Building a Community School. New York: Author; 1997.

[23] McKnight J. The Careless Society: Community and its Counterfeits. New York: Basic
      Books, 1995.

[24] Osher TW, deFur E, Nava C, Spencer S, Toth-Dennis D. New Roles for Families in
      Systems of Care. Washington, DC: American Institutes of Research, Center for Effec-
      tive Collaboration and Practice; 1999.

[25] Bennett J, Grimly LK. Parenting in the Global Community. A Cross-Cultural/Interna-
      tional Perspective. In Fine M, Lee S. (eds.) Handbook of Diversity in Parent Educa-
      tion: The Changing Faces of Parenting and Parent Education. San Diego, CA:
      Academic Press; 2001, p96-132.

[26] Fristad MA, Goldberg-Arnold JS, Gavazzi SM. Multi-Family Psychoeducation
      Groups in the Treatment of Children with Mood Disorders. Journal of Marital Family
      Therapy 2003;29(4) 491-504.

[27] Duchanowski AJ, Kurash K, Friedman RM. Community-Based Interventions in a
      System of Care and Outcomes of Framework. In Burns BJ, Hoagwood K. (eds.) Com-
      munity Treatment for Youth: Evidence-Based Interventions for Severe Emotional and
      Behavioral Disorders. New York: Oxford University Press; 2002, p16-38.

[28] Friesen BJ, Huff B. Family Perspectives on Systems of Care. In Stroul B. (ed.) Chil-
      dren's Mental Health: Creating Systems of Care in a Changing Society. Baltimore:
      Paul H. Brookes; 1996, p41-67.

[29] Ruffolo MC, Kuhn MT, Evans ME. Developing a Parent-Professional Team Leader-
      ship Model in Group Work: Work with Families with Children Experiencing Behav-
      ioral and Emotional Problems. Social Work 2006;51(1) 39-47.

[30] Bruner C. Thinking Collaboratively: Ten Questions and Answers to Help Policy
      Makers Improve Children's Services. Washington, DC: Education and Human Serv-
      ices Consortium; 1991.

[31] Cunningham CC, Davis H. Early Parenting Counseling. In Craft M, Bichnell J, Hollins S. (eds.) Mental Handicap: A Multidisciplinary Approach. London: Bailliere Tindall; 1985, p69-88.

[32] Marteau TM, Johnston M, Baum JD, Bloch S. Goals of Treatment in Diabetes: A Comparison of Doctors and Parents of Children with Diabetes. Journal of Behavioral Medicine1987;10(1) 33-48.

[33] Betz M, O'Connell L. Changing Doctor-Patient Relationships and the Rise in Concern for Accountability. Social Problems 1983;31(1) 84-95.

[34] Pugh G, De'Ath E. Working Towards Partnership in Early Years. London: National Children's Bureau; 1989.

[35] Mittler P, McConachie H. Parents, Professionals and Mentally Handicapped People: Approaches to Partnership. Beckenham: Croom Helm; 1983.

[36] Mittler P, Mittler H. The Transitional Relationship. In Mittler P, McConachie H. (eds.) Parents, Professionals and Mentally Handicapped People: Approaches to Partnership. Beckenham: Croom Helm; 1983, p221-240.

[37] Turnbull AP, Turnbull HR. Parent Involvement in the Education of Handicapped Children: A Critique. Mental Retardation1982;20(2) 115-122.

[38] Davis PB, May JE. Involving Fathers in Early Intervention and Family Support Programs: Issues and Strategies. Child Health Care 1991;20(1) 87-92.

[39] Appleton PL, Minchom PE. Models of Parent Partnership and Child Development Centers. Child: Care, Health and Development 1991;17(1) 27-38.

[40] Dale P. Parent Report Assessment of Language and Communication. In Cole K, Dale P, Thal D. (eds.) Assessment of Communication and Language. Baltimore, MD: Paul H. Brookes; 1996, p161-182.

[41] McConkey R. Working with Parents: A Practical Guide for Teachers and Therapists. London: Croom Helm; 1986.

[42] New C, David M. For the Children's Sake: Making Childcare More than Women's Business. Harmondsworth: Penguin; 1985.

[43] Ayer S, Alaszewski A. Community Care and the Mentally Handicapped: Services for Mothers and their Mentally Handicapped Children. London: Croom Helm; 1984.

[44] Glendenning C. Parents and their Disabled Children. London: Routledge and Kegan Paul; 1983.

[45] Feinberg E, Vacca J. The Drama and the Trauma of Creating Policies on Autism: Critical Issues to Consider in the New Millennium. Focus on Autism and Other Developmental Disabilities 2000;15(2) 130-138.

[46] Hannam C. Parents and Mentally Handicapped Children. Harmondsworth: Penguin; 1975.

[47] Quine L, Rutter DR. First Diagnosis of Severe Mental and Physical Disability: A Study of Doctor-Patient Communication. Journal of Child Psychology and Psychiatry 1994;35(7) 1273-1287.

[48] Friend M, Cook L. Interactions: Collaborative Skills for School Professionals. White Plains, NY: Longman; 1992.

[49] Fine MJ. The Handbook of Family-School Intervention: A Systems Perspective. Boston: Allyn & Bacon; 1991.

[50] Kalyva E. Autism: Educational and Therapeutic Approaches. London: Sage; 2011.

[51] Hecimovic A, Gregory S. The Evolving Role, Impact, and Needs of Families. In Zager D. (ed.) Autism Spectrum Disorders: Identification, Education, and Treatment. 3rd ed. Mahwah, NJ: Lawrence Erlbaum Associates; 2005, p111-142.

[52] Lovaas OI. Behavioral Treatment and Normal Educational and Intellectual Functioning in Young Autistic Children. Journal of Consulting and Clinical Psychology 1987;5(1) 3-9.

[53] Schopler E, Mesibov GB, Hearsey KA. Structured Teaching in the TEACCH System. In Schopler E, Mesibov GB. (eds.), Learning and Cognition in Autism. New York: Plenum; 1995, p243-268.

[54] Hardy N, Sturmey P. Portage Guide to Early Education, III: A Rapid Training and Feedback System to Teach and Maintain Mothers' Teaching Skills. Educational Psychology 1994;14(3) 345-358.

[55] Ruble LA, Dalrymple NJ. COMPASS: A Parent-Teacher Collaborative Model for Students with Autism. Focus on Autism and Other Developmental Disabilities 2002;17(1) 76-83.

[56] Friesen BJ. Creating Change for Children with Serious Emotional Disorders: A National Strategy. In Mizrahi T, Morrison J. (eds.). Community Organizations and Social Administration: Advances, Trends and Emerging Principles. New York: Haworth Press; 1993, p127-146.

[57] Kohler F. Examining the Services Received by Young Children with Autism and their Families: A Survey of Parent Responses. Focus on Autism and Other Developmental Disabilities 1999;14(2) 150-158.

[58] Johnson HC. Family Issues and Interventions. In Johnson HC. (ed.) Child Mental Health in the 1990s: Curricula for Graduate and Undergraduate Professional Education. Washington, DC: U.S. Department of Health and Human Services, Public Health Service, National Institute of Mental Health; 1993, p85-101.

[59] Read J, Clements L. Disabled Children and the Law: Research, the Law and Good Practice. London: Jessica Kingsley Publishers; 2001.

[60] Soodak LC, Erwin EJ, Winton P, et al. Implementing Inclusive Early Childhood Education: A Call for Professional Empowerment. Topics in Early Childhood Special Education 2002;22(1) 91-102.

[61] Collins B, Collins T. Parent-Professional Relationships in the Treatment of Seriously Emotionally Disturbed Children and Adolescents. Social Work 1990;35(5) 522-527.

[62] Smith DE, Griffith AI. Coordinating the Uncoordinated: Mothering, Schooling and the Family Wage. Perspectives of Social Problems 1990;2(1) 25-43.

[63] Crawford T, Simonoff E. Parental Views about Services for Children Attending Schools for the Emotionally and Behaviourally Disturbed (EBD): A Qualitative Analysis. Child: Care, Health and Development 2003;29(6) 481-491.

[64] Francell C, Conn V, Gray D. Families' Perceptions of Burden of Care for Chronic Mentally Ill Relatives. Hospital of Community Psychology 1988;39(12) 1296-1937.

[65] Tarico V, Low B, Trupin E, Forsyth-Stephens A. Children's Mental Health Services: A Parent Perspective. Community and Mental Health Journal 1989;25(3) 313-326.

[66] Johnson HC, Renaud E. Professional Beliefs about Parents of Children with Mental and Emotional Disabilities: A Cross-Discipline Comparison. Journal of Emotional and Behavioral Disorders 1995;5(2) 149-161.

[67] Randall P, Parker J. Supporting the Families of Children with Autism. Chichester: Wiley; 1999.

[68] Hartman A, Laird J. Family-Centered Social Work Practice. New York: Free Press; 1983.

[69] Bennett WS, Hokenstad MC. Full-Time People Workers and Conceptions of the Professional. In Halmos P, (ed.) Professionalism and Social Change. Keele: University of Keele Press; 1973, p36-58.

[70] Handy CB. Understanding Organizations. Harmondsworth: Penguin; 1985.

[71] Cone JD, Delawyer DD, Wolfe VV. Assessing Parent Participation: The Parent/Family Involvement Index. Exceptional Children 1985;51(3) 417-424.

[72] Smets AC. Family and Staff Attitudes toward Family Involvement in the Treatment of Hospitalized Chronic Patients. Hospital Community Psychiatry 1982;33(6) 573-575.

[73] Brand S. Making Parent Involvement a Reality: Helping Teachers Develop Partnerships with Parents. Young Children 1996;51(1) 76-81.

[74] Katz L, Bauch J. The Peabody family involvement initiative: Preparing preservice teachers for family/school collaboration. The School Community Journal 1999;9(1) 49-69.

[75] Tichenor M. Teacher Education and Parent Involvement: Reflections from Preservice Teachers. Journal of Instructional Psychology 1997;24(2) 233-240.

[76] Dinnebeil LA, Hale LM, Rule S. A Qualitative Analysis of Parents' and Service Coordinators' Descriptions of Variables that Influence Collaborative Relationships. Topics in Early Childhood Special Education 1996:19(4) 322-347.

[77] Dunst CJ, Trivette CM, Johanson C. Parent-Professional Collaboration and Partnership. In Dunst CJ, Trivette CM, Deal AG. (eds.) Supporting and Strengthening Families. Cambridge, MA: Brookline Books; 1994, p197-211.

[78] Summers JA, Hoffman L, Marquis J, Turnbull A, Poston D, Lord Nelson L. Measuring the Quality of Family-Professional Partnerships in Special Education Services. Exceptional Children 2005;72(1) 65-81.

[79] Stevenson O, Parsloe P. Community Care and Empowerment. York. Joseph Rowntree Foundation; 1993.

[80] Loxley A. Collaboration in Health and Welfare: Working with Difference. London. Jessica Kingsley Publishers; 1997.

[81] Malin N. Services for People with Learning Disabilities. London: Routledge; 1995.

[82] Goble R. Multi-Professional Education in Europe. In Leathard A, (ed.) Going Inter-Professional: Working Together for Health and Welfare. London: Routledge; 1994, p157-194.

[83] Wistow G. Hospital Discharge and Community Care: Early Days. Leeds: Nuffield Institute for Health; 1993.

[84] Roberts RN, Rule S, Innocenti MS. Strengthening the Family-Professional Partnership in Services for Young Children. Baltimore: Brookes; 1998.

[85] Epstein JL. School, Family, and Community Partnership: Preparing Educators and Improving Schools. Boulder, CO: Westview Press; 2001.

[86] Osher TW, Osher DM. The Paradigm Shift to True Collaboration with Families. Journal of Child and Family Studies 2002;11(1) 47-60.

[87] Bruder MB. Family-Centered Early Intervention: Clarifying our Values for the New Millennium. Topics in Early Childhood Special Education 2000;20(1) 105-115.

[88] Trivette CM, Dunst CJ, Boyd K, Hamby D. Family-Oriented Program Models, Help Giving Practices, and Parental Control Appraisals. Exceptional Children 1995;62(2) 237-248.

[89] Applequist KL, Bailey DB. Navajo Caregivers' Perceptions of Early Intervention Services. Journal of Early Intervention Services 2000;23(1) 47-61.

[90] McWilliam RA, Tocci L, Harbin GL. Family-Centered Services: Service Providers' Discourse and Behavior. Topics in Early Childhood Special Education 1998;18(2) 206-221.

[91] Park J, Turnbull AP. Service Integration in Early Intervention: Determining Interpersonal and Structural Factors for its Success. Infants and Young Children 2003;16(1) 48-58.

[92] Parette HP, Brotherson MJ, Huer MB. (2000). Giving Families a Voice in Augmentative and Alternative Communication Decision-Making. Education and Training in Mental Retardation and Developmental Disabilities 2000;35(2) 77-90.

[93] Soodak L, Erwin E. Valued Member or Tolerated Participant: Parents' Experiences in Inclusive Early Childhood Settings. Journal of the Association of Parents with Severe Handicaps 2000;25(1) 29-41.

[94] Park J, Turnbull AP. Families Speak Out: What are Quality Indicators of Professionals in Working with Children with Problem Behavior? Journal of Positive Behavioral Intervention 2002;4(2) 118-123.

[95] McWilliam R, Maxwell K, Sloper K. Beyond Involvement: Are Elementary Schools Ready to be Family Centered? School Psychology Review 1999;28(3) 378-394.

[96] Rainforth B, York J, Macdonald C. Collaborative Teams for Students with Severe Disabilities: Integrating Therapy and Educational Services. Baltimore: Brooks; 1992.

[97] Salembier GB, Furney KS. Speaking up for your Child's Future. Exceptional Parent 1998;28(1) 62-64.

[98] Sanders M. Improving School, Family and Community Partnerships in Urban Middle Schools. Middle School Journal 1999;31(1): 35-41.

[99] Blue-Banning MJ, Turnbull AP, Pereira L. Group Action Planning as a Support Strategy for Hispanic Families: Parent and Professional Perspectives. Mental Retardation 2000;38(2) 262-275.

[100] Allen RL, Perry CG. Toward Developing Standards and Measurements for Family-Centered Practice in Family Support Programs. In Singer GHS, Powers LE, Olson AL. (ed.) Redefining Family Support: Innovations in Public-Private Partnerships. Baltimore: Brookes; 1996. p57-86.

[101] Dunst CJ. Revisiting "Rethinking Early Intervention". Topics in Early Childhood Special Education 2000;20(1) 95-104.

[102] Kalyanpur M, Harry B. Culture in Special Education. Baltimore: Brookes; 1999.

[103] Lynch EW, Hanson MJ. Developing Cross-Cultural Competence: A Guide for Working with Children and Families. 2nd ed. Baltimore: Brookes; 1998.

[104] Sileo TW, Prater MA. Preparing Professionals for Partnerships with Parents of Students with Disabilities: Textbook Considerations Regarding Cultural Diversity. Exceptional Children 1998;64(5) 513-528.

[105] Blue-Banning MJ, Summers JA, Frankland C, Nelson LGL, Beegle G. Dimensions of Parent-Professional Partnerships. Exceptional Children 2004;70(1) 167-184.

[106] Lord Nelson LG, Summers JA, Turnbull AP. Boundaries in Family-Professional Relationships. Remedial and Special Education 2004;25(3) 153-165.

[107] Ruble L, Sears L. Diagnostic Assessment of Autistic Disorder. In Huebner R. (ed.) Autism and Related Disorders: A Sensorimotor Approach to Management. Maryland: Aspen; 2000, p41-59.

[108] Ruble LA, Dalrymple NJ. An Alternative View of Outcome in Autism. Focus on Autism and Other Developmental Disabilities 1996;11(1) 3-14.

[109] McWilliam R, Young H, Harville K. Satisfaction and Struggles: Family Perceptions of Early Intervention Services. Journal of Early Intervention 1995;19(1) 43-60.

[110] Murphy DL, Lee IM, Turnbull AP, Turbiville V. The Family-Centered Program Rating Scale: An Instrument for Program Evaluation and Changes. Journal of Early Intervention 1995;19(1) 24-42.

[111] McNaughton D. Measuring Parent Satisfaction with Early Childhood Intervention Programs: Current Practice, Problems, and Future Perspectives. Topics in Early Childhood Special Education 1994;10(1) 1-15.

[112] Lake JF, Billingsley BS. An Analysis of Factors that Contribute to Parent-School Conflict in Special Education. Remedial and Special Education 2000;21(4) 240-251.

[113] Minke K, Scott M. Parent Professional Relationships in Early Intervention: A Qualitative Investigation. Topics in Early Childhood Special Education 1995;15(3) 335-346.

[114] Dominique B, Cuttler B, McTarnaghan J. The Experience of Autism in the Lives of Families. In Wetherby AM, Prizant BM. (eds). Autism Spectrum Disorders: A Transactional Developmental Perspective. Baltimore: Brooks; 2000, p369-394.

[115] Lambie R. Working with Families of at Risk and Special Needs Students: A Systems Change Model. Focus on Exceptional Children 2000;32(1) 1-22.

[116] Powers M. Children with Autism: A Parent's Guide. 2nd ed. Bethesda, MD: Woodbine House; 2000.

[117] Katz L. Dispositions: Definitions and Implications for Early Childhood Practices. New York: ERIC; 1993.

[118] Stoner JB, Bock SJ, Thompson JR, Angell ME, Heyl BS, Crowley EP. Welcome to our World: Parent Perceptions of Interactions between Parents of Young Children with ASD and Education Professionals. Focus on Autism and Other Developmental Disabilities 2005;20(1) 39-51.

[119] Bartolo PA. Communicating a Diagnosis of Developmental Disability to Parents: Multiprofessional Negotiation Frameworks. Child: Care, Health and Development 2002;28(1) 65-71.

[120] Buckman R, Kason Y. How to Break Bad News: A Practical Protocol for Health Professionals. London: Macmillan; 1992.

[121] Siegel B. Coping with the Diagnosis of Autism. In Cohen DJ, Volkmar FR. (eds.) Handbook of Autism and Pervasive Developmental Disorders. New York: Wiley; 1997, p460-483.

[122] Cottrell DJ, Summers K. Communicating an Evolutionary Diagnosis of Disability to Parents. Child: Care, Health and Development 1990;16(2) 211-218.

[123] Cohen DJ, Volkmar FR. Handbook of Autism and Pervasive Developmental Disorders. New York: Wiley; 1997.

[124] Freeman WJ. Neurohumoral Brain Dynamics of Social Group Formation: Implications for Autism. In Carter CH, Lederhendler H, Kirkpatrick B. (eds.) The Integrative Neurobiology of Affiliation. New York: Annals of the New York Academy of Sciences; 1997, p501-503.

[125] Abrams EZ, Goodman JF. Diagnosing Developmental Problems in Children: Parents and Professionals Negotiate Bad News. Journal of Pediatric Psychology 1998; 23(1) 87-98.

[126] Gill VT, Maynard DW. On "Labelling" in Actual Interaction: Delivering and Receiving Diagnoses of Developmental Disabilities. Social Problems 1995;42(1) 11-37.

[127] Maynard DW. Bearing Bad News in Clinical Settings. In Dervin B. (ed.) Progress in Communication Sciences. Norwood, N.J.: Ablex; 1991, p143-172.

[128] Bailey D, Scarborough A, Hebbeler K. Families' First Experiences with Early Intervention. Menlo Park, CA: SRI International; 2003.

[129] King G, King S, Rosenbaum P, Goffin R. Family-Centered Caregiving and Well-Being of Parents of Children with Disabilities. Journal of Pediatric Psychology 1999;24(1) 41-53.

[130] Thompson L, Lobb C, Elling R, Herman S, Jurkiewicz T, Hulleza C. Pathways to Family Empowerment: Effects of Family-Centered Delivery of Early Intervention Services. Exceptional Children 1997;64(1) 99-113.

[131] Laws G, Millward L. Predicting Parents' Satisfaction with the Education of their Child with Down Syndrome. Education Research 2001;43(2) 209-226.

[132] Rao SS. Perspectives of an African American Mother on Parent-Professional Relationships in Special Education. Mental Retardation 2000;38(3) 475-488.

[133] Park J, Turnbull AP. Cross-Cultural Competency and Special Education: Perception and Experiences of Korean Parents of Children with Special Needs. Education and Training in Mental Retardation and Developmental Disabilities 2001;36(2) 133-147.

[134] Able-Boone H, Goodwin I, Sandall S, Gordon N, Martin D. Consumer-Based Early Intervention Services. Journal of Early Intervention 1992;16(2) 201-209.

[135] Covert SB. Whatever it Takes! Excellence in Family Support: When Families Experience a Disability. St. Augustine, FL: Training Resource Network, Inc; 1995.

[136] Karp D. Speaking of Sadness: Depression, Disconnection, and the Meanings of Illness. Oxford: Oxford University Press; 1996.

[137] Goldstein H. On Boundaries. Family and Society – Journal of Contemporary History 1999;80(5) 435-438.

[138] Strom-Gottfied, K. Professional Boundaries: An Analysis of Violations by Social Workers. Family and Society – Journal of Contemporary History 1999;80(4) 439-449.

[139] British Psychological Society. Code of Ethics and Conduct. Leicester: Author; 2009.

[140] American Psychiatric Association. Diagnostic and Statistical Manual for Mental Disorders. 4th ed. text revision. Washington, DC: American Psychiatric Association; 2000.

[141] Health and Care Professions Council. Fitness to Practice. http://www.hpc-uk.org/aboutus/committees/ftp/ (accessed 15 June 2008).

[142] Cournoyer DE, Johnson HC. Measuring Parents' Perceptions of Mental Health Professionals. Research in Social Work and Practice 1991;1(3) 399-415.

[143] Johnson HC, Cournoyer DE. Measuring Worker Cognitions about Parents of Children with Mental and Emotional Disabilities. Journal of Emotional and Behavioral Disorders 1994;2(1) 99-108.

[144] Darling RB, Baxter C. Families in Focus: Socio-Logical Methods in Early Intervention. Austin, TX: Pro-Ed; 1996.

[145] Gowen JW, Christy DS, Sparling J. Informational Needs of Parents of Young Children with Special Needs. Journal of Early Intervention 1993;17(2) 194-210.

[146] Hassall R, Rose J, McDonald J. Parenting Stress in Mothers of Children with an Intellectual Disability: The Effects of Parental Cognitions in Relation to Child Characteristics and Family Support. Journal of Intellectual Disability Research 2005;49(6) 405-418.

[147] Summers JA, Gavin K, Hall T, Nelson J. Family and School Partnerships: Building Bridges in General and Special Education. In Obiakor FE, Utley A, Rotatori AF. (eds.). Advances in Special Education: Psychology of Effective Education for Learners with Exceptionalities. Stamford, CT: JAI Press; 2003, p417-445.

[148] Muscott HS. Exceptional Partnerships: Listening to the Voices of Families. Preventing School Failure 2002;42(1) 66-69.

[149] Dillenburger K, Keenan M, Gallagher S, McElhinney M. Parent Education and Home-Based Behaviour Analytic Intervention: An Examination of Parents' Perceptions and Emotions. Journal of Intellectual and Developmental Disabilities 2004;29(1) 119-130.

[150] Longenecker H. Parental Stress - ABA and Traditional Special Education Programs. http://rsaffran.tripod.com/longenecker.html. (accessed 28 June 2006).

[151] Laborde PR, Seligman M. Counseling Parents with Children with Disabilities. In Se-
       ligman M. (ed.) The Family with a Handicapped Child. 2nd ed. Boston: Allyn & Ba-
       con; 1991, p337-369.

[152] Moscovici S. Social Change and Influence. London: Academic Press; 1978.

[153] Field S, Hoffman A. The Importance of Family Involvement for Promoting Self-De-
       termination in Adolescents with Autism and Other Developmental Disabilities. Fo-
       cus on Autism and Other Developmental Disabilities 1999;14(1) 36-41.

[154] Renty J, Roeyers H. Quality of Life in High-Functioning Adults with Autism Spec-
       trum Disorder: The Predictive Value of Disability and Support Characteristics. Au-
       tism 2006;10(5) 511-524.

[155] Avramidis E, Kalyva E. Research Methods in Special Needs: Theory and Practice.
       Athens: Papazisis; 2006.

[156] Kalantzi-Azizi A, Besevengkis E. Issues of Training and Sensitization of Mental
       Health Professionals Working with Children and Adolescents; 2000.

Permissions

The contributors of this book come from diverse backgrounds, making this book a truly international effort. This book will bring forth new frontiers with its revolutionizing research information and detailed analysis of the nascent developments around the world.

We would like to thank Professor Michael Fitzgerald, for lending his expertise to make the book truly unique. He has played a crucial role in the development of this book. Without his invaluable contribution this book wouldn't have been possible. He has made vital efforts to compile up to date information on the varied aspects of this subject to make this book a valuable addition to the collection of many professionals and students.

This book was conceptualized with the vision of imparting up-to-date information and advanced data in this field. To ensure the same, a matchless editorial board was set up. Every individual on the board went through rigorous rounds of assessment to prove their worth. After which they invested a large part of their time researching and compiling the most relevant data for our readers. Conferences and sessions were held from time to time between the editorial board and the contributing authors to present the data in the most comprehensible form. The editorial team has worked tirelessly to provide valuable and valid information to help people across the globe.

Every chapter published in this book has been scrutinized by our experts. Their significance has been extensively debated. The topics covered herein carry significant findings which will fuel the growth of the discipline. They may even be implemented as practical applications or may be referred to as a beginning point for another development. Chapters in this book were first published by InTech; hereby published with permission under the Creative Commons Attribution License or equivalent.

The editorial board has been involved in producing this book since its inception. They have spent rigorous hours researching and exploring the diverse topics which have resulted in the successful publishing of this book. They have passed on their knowledge of decades through this book. To expedite this challenging task, the publisher supported the team at every step. A small team of assistant editors was also appointed to further simplify the editing procedure and attain best results for the readers.

Our editorial team has been hand-picked from every corner of the world. Their multi-ethnicity adds dynamic inputs to the discussions which result in innovative outcomes. These outcomes are then further discussed with the researchers and contributors who give their valuable feedback and opinion regarding the same. The feedback is then collaborated with the researches and they are edited in a comprehensive manner to aid the understanding of the subject.

Apart from the editorial board, the designing team has also invested a significant amount of their time in understanding the subject and creating the most relevant covers. They scrutinized every image to scout for the most suitable representation of the subject and create an appropriate cover for the book.

The publishing team has been involved in this book since its early stages. They were actively engaged in every process, be it collecting the data, connecting with the contributors or procuring relevant information. The team has been an ardent support to the editorial, designing and production team. Their endless efforts to recruit the best for this project, has resulted in the accomplishment of this book. They are a veteran in the field of academics and their pool of knowledge is as vast as their experience in printing. Their expertise and guidance has proved useful at every step. Their uncompromising quality standards have made this book an exceptional effort. Their encouragement from time to time has been an inspiration for everyone.

The publisher and the editorial board hope that this book will prove to be a valuable piece of knowledge for researchers, students, practitioners and scholars across the globe.

List of Contributors

Jenny Fairthorne, Amanda Langridge, Jenny Bourke and Helen Leonard
Centre for Child Health, University of Western Australia, Australia

Ginny Russell
University of Exeter Medical School, ESRC Centre for Genomics in Society, UK

Zsuzsa Pavelka
University of Milan, Italy

Maria R. Urbano, Kathrin Hartmann, Stephen I. Deutsch,
Gina M. Bondi Polychronopoulos and Vanessa Dorbin
Department of Psychiatry and Behavioral Sciences, Eastern Virginia Medical School, Norfolk, Virginia, USA

Gitta De Vaan, Mathijs P.J. Vervloed, and Ludo Verhoeven
Behavioural Science Institute, Radboud University Nijmegen, Nijmegen The Netherlands, Royal Kentalis, Sint-Michielsgestel, The Netherlands

Harry Knoors
Behavioural Science Institute, Radboud University Nijmegen, Nijmegen The Netherlands, Royal Kentalis, Sint-Michielsgestel, The Netherlands

Kieran D. O'Malley
Charlemont Clinic/ Our Lady's Children's Hospital Crumlin, Dublin, Ireland

Jennifer Elder
University of Florida College of Nursing, Gainesville, Florida, USA

Efrosini Kalyva
Psychology Department, The International Faculty of the University of Sheffield, CITY College, Thessaloniki, Greece

Printed in the USA
CPSIA information can be obtained
at www.ICGtesting.com
JSHW011405221024
72173JS00003B/429